What Snack Girl Readers Have to Say

"Just wanted to tell you that I have made several of your recipes with tremendous success. I am not someone who ever loved to cook but in my quest to eat healthier, I realized I must learn and you offer so many great variations of foods that are usually on my 'don't' list. The recipes actually get me excited about cooking (which is very shocking to friends, family, and my husband)."

—Ilyse, New Providence, New Jersey

"I'm absolutely enjoying your advice and guidance; always informative and thought provoking. Snack Girl is very helpful on my weight loss journey. I joined Weight Watchers in January of this year and have lost a little over 30 pounds and am about 17 pounds from goal. Thank you for all you do in supporting a healthy lifestyle. Your daily post keeps me motivated and inspired. I look forward to opening my daily dose of Snack Girl over coffee each morning."

—Sydney, Monterey, California

"Your research, humor, and straightforward approach have made me an instant fan! I've shared your blog with other friends who care about great food, nutrition, and all the things in between. You deserve a crown of gold stars!"

—Mary, Charlottesville, Virginia

"I work at Costco and I come in contact with many, many people who are trying to adopt a healthier lifestyle. I must tell you that I tell everyone who is interested about how wonderful your site is! I know that they will enjoy it as much as I do. Thank you."

—Robin, Buford, Georgia

"I am loving your daily e-mails and tips. I like that you feature 'normal' food and yet introduce me to new stuff as I am becoming a healthy new me! Thanks for your awesome information!"

—Tammie, Alexandria, Minnesota

"Before Snack Girl came into my life, I was a zombie walking down each aisle of the grocery store, falling for advertising gimmicks that promised whole grain or real fruit juice or no sugar added. But now, because of Snack Girl, I am oh so aware of the ingredients in products and the games manufacturers play to get our attention. You explain things so well and I am thankful for you. Thank you for being a wonderful voice and guide to be a healthy active mother and wife."

—Jessica, Riverdale, Utah

"I love your e-mail updates! I have never been a 'good' eater and Snack Girl is making me much more aware of what I am eating. I am enjoying healthier foods. Thank you!"

—Marcy, Lowville, New York

"I rejoined Weight Watchers recently—tenth time is the charm, isn't it?—and realize part of the problem I've had in the last few attempts was having to eat so differently from the rest of the family. (And the rest of the world, it felt like!) Your suggestions are quick, easy, and yummy."

—Cathy, Nova Scotia, Canada

"I just wanted to drop you a quick note to tell you how much I appreciate your e-mails and information. I studied nutrition in college but needed to be reinspired. My husband caught me the other day yelping out 'I love you Snack Girl!'"

—Patricia, Cape Fear, North Carolina

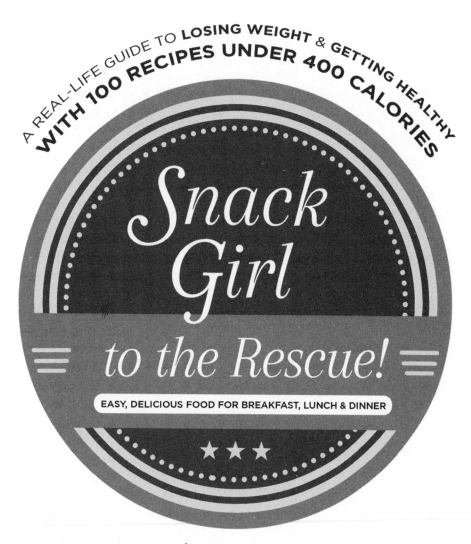

A REAL-LIFE GUIDE TO LOSING WEIGHT & GETTING HEALTHY

WITH 100 RECIPES UNDER 400 CALORIES

Snack Girl
to the Rescue!

EASY, DELICIOUS FOOD FOR BREAKFAST, LUNCH & DINNER

★ ★ ★

LISA CAIN

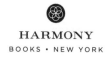

HARMONY

BOOKS • NEW YORK

Copyright © 2014 by Lisa Cain
Published in the United States by Harmony Books, an imprint of the Crown
Publishing Group, a division of Random House LLC, a Penguin Random House
Company, New York. www.crownpublishing.com

Harmony Books is a registered trademark, and the Circle colophon
is a trademark of Random House LLC.

Some of the recipes and information in this book have appeared, in different
form, on the author's website, Snack-Girl.com.

Library of Congress Cataloging-in-Publication Data
Cain, Lisa, 1969–
Snack Girl to the rescue!: a real life guide to eating healthy, slimming down, and
enjoying food/Lisa Cain.—First edition.
pages cm
1. Reducing diets—Recipes. 2. Reducing exercises. 3. Health. 4. Nutrition. I.
Title.
RM222.2.C224 2013
613.2'5—dc2   2013020382

ISBN 978-0-385-34908-6
Ebook ISBN 978-0-385-34909-3

Printed in the United States of America

Book design by Maria Elias and Elizabeth Rendfleisch
Illustration on page 26 courtesy of the National Heart, Lung, and Blood Institute
Cover design by Nupoor Gordon
Cover illustration by Kirsten Ulve

10   9   8   7   6   5   4   3   2   1
First Edition

For Matt, Ruby, and Alex, my whole enchilada

Contents

PART 2

Recipes

Introduction

Do you need to be rescued from the diet roller coaster or junk food? I'm guessing if you are looking at this page, you probably need some help. I'm glad you picked up this book because I, Snack Girl, am here to lift you up with encouragement, practical advice, recipes, a little humor, and a lot of love. My website, Snack-Girl.com, has thousands of readers every day who get inspired to change what they eat. If we can do it, you can too.

Before Snack Girl: How I Began My Journey

When I was in my twenties, I ate whatever I wanted and I looked and felt great. I had joined the dot-com boom in San Francisco, and had the luxury of biking to and from work every day. The office buildings were filled with people who loved to throw a Frisbee at lunch and would go on eight-mile hikes on the weekend. I was *so* active that I hardly ever packed my lunch or cooked a meal; I just ordered whatever my compatriots were eating (burritos, doughnuts, pizza) and enjoyed it. The mantra at the time was "Work hard, play hard." I never read a food label, gave a damn about saturated fat, or thought about the origin of my produce.

The dot-com crash burst my personal bubble and I was out of a job three times in a two-year period. I kept getting laid off as each company that I joined failed for a variety of reasons. After I was humiliated (yet again) when a security guard stood by as I cleaned out my desk, I decided that I needed to focus on some other life goals, because my career was in a nosedive.

Right at this moment of career crisis, I met a sweet Australian and we fell in love. He surprised me by asking me to marry him and we decided to have a family. Our plans were for both of us to continue working and have a few rug rats. Ruby arrived about a year after we were married and I was so in love with her that I didn't want to go back to work. Fortunately, our finances allowed me to stay home and I began a life of diapers, laundry, and insufficient sleep. I was exhausted and, other than pushing a stroller up a hill, daily exercise was no longer part of my routine.

Did I feel like getting a gym membership? Heck, no! I spent most of my time dreaming of a hotel room with a comfy bed. In my dream, the white bed was made and all I had to do was change into my (free of breast milk stains) soft jammies, put my head on the pillow, and sleep. Alone. I thought about this *a lot* my first year of motherhood.

We added rug rat number two, Alex, two years later. Alex's first year of life is a blur. Needless to say, I have since apologized to my husband for my behavior for the *entire year*. Yes, I was grumpy, demanding, and difficult. I did my best to nurture my children and did a lousy job of nurturing myself. I loved being a mother, but I was ill suited for all the interruptions, messy meals, crying, naps, and general chaos that having children brings.

About a year after Alex was born, my doctor's office called to remind me that it was time for my physical and, in a move to start taking care of my health, I scheduled an appointment. There, as I sat on the edge of the examining table, my kind doctor looked me straight in the eye and said, "We need to talk about your weight."

I panicked. "My weight?"

"Lisa, you need to lose weight. You are increasing your risk factors for a bunch of diseases and if you keep adding pounds like this, you will become obese."

How could I be having this conversation? Yeah, I was carrying around some extra weight, but I kept thinking it would magically come off.

I wanted to shout, "It's my kids—they won't let me sleep! It's the doughnut place around the corner! I just need a gym membership! I just *can't* give up the cream in my coffee!"

I said, "Okay, I'll work on it." I left his office with my chin dragging on the ground.

What was I going to do? My love affair with Food is a long one and I didn't want to change it. We are so good together, Food and I. When I was sad, bored, or lonely, Food was there to lift me up. When it was time to celebrate, Food and I had a great time.

What was I going to do without Food? Sniff.

On the other hand, my children, Ruby and Alex, instilled in me a burning desire to live for as long as I could. I love their smell, their laugh, and their little hands in mine—for me, the closest thing to heaven on earth.

Also, I didn't feel very good. I had no energy and I always felt like I wanted a nap. I couldn't stay up past 9 p.m. and when I walked up the steep hills of San Francisco, I felt winded after a few steps. Sometimes I was so tired that I would count the hours until my children went to sleep. "Three hours to go!" I would think and just try to get to 8 p.m. without losing my temper. I was eating mega cookies or cupcakes every day at 3 p.m. with a large double-shot latte to stay awake, then crashing at 5 p.m. when the sugar had left my system. I blamed this on my children's habit of waking me in the night, but the truth is that extra pounds take more energy to carry around.

My doctor was telling me what I didn't want to hear. That time of my life when I could do what I wanted and consequences be damned was over, baby.

I approached the problem like the trained scientist that I am. Though I was now a stay-at-home mom, I had earned a PhD in genetics in 1997 and had quit science to join the Internet revolution.

First, I started dieting and read every diet book I could get my hands on. I found the conflicting messages in the books confusing. Many of the books seemed to be advocating extreme approaches to food. For example, there was the no-carbohydrate approach. Ummm, I don't want to spend my life without rice, pasta, or bread.

Or there was a quick-weight-loss strategy where I would consume only 1,000 calories per day (the FDA recommends an average of 2,000 calories for an adult). How was I going to do that and not become incredibly irritable? If I get too hungry, I start to act like a crazy person, and no one wants to see that.

Going vegan was another route. I can see how giving up all animal products could lead to significant weight loss, but my toes curl at the scent of bacon. Couldn't I just eat less meat?

So many of these diets seemed faddish and ultimately unhealthy. They were asking me for sacrifices that were, in my mind, unreasonable. They promised me quick results, but I wanted sustainable weight loss that would help protect me from developing cancer, diabetes, and heart disease. Looking good in my clothes again, having more energy, and just feeling good were also priorities.

My parents had recently lost 70 pounds combined on Weight Watchers and were both convinced that this was the best approach. My mother had just retired from her high-pressure job and decided that she was finally going to tackle her weight problem. She got my dad to join her and they were bubbling over about the program. It felt like every day they were calling me with a new victory over the scale. But they lived five hours away in Los Angeles, which meant I was going to have to go it alone in San Francisco.

I attended my first Weight Watchers meeting in an upscale part of town and found myself stepping on a scale surrounded by a group of twenty-something thin people in Spandex gym clothes. Uh-oh.

The leader started by talking about Thanksgiving and how she had managed to eat a mere one ounce of turkey with her family in South Dakota. She kept talking about all the food she skipped that I am sure someone lovingly prepared. I started to sweat. When was she going to stop talking about marshmallow-covered sweet potatoes and pecan pie?

I wanted to shout, "Hey, lady, next time you go to Thanksgiving, could you bring me a few foil-wrapped plates of all that lovely food you avoided?"

When the meeting ended, I ran out the door to my car, drove home, and cried. My halfhearted attempts at weight loss using a low-carb diet, going vegan, food journaling, and Weight Watchers were leading me nowhere. I was exhausted from trying so hard, and every time I lost weight I gained it right back. I was beginning to hate how I felt and looked. I needed a new approach.

The Snack Girl Life Plan Is Born

I did what every self-respecting mother of two small children would do in this situation. I quit. I simply couldn't juggle all my responsibilities and successfully attempt any of the diets that I had researched. It was futile for me to keep trying, so I gave up.

My first piece of advice for anyone trying hard but failing to lose weight?

Give up! Yes, dear reader, I want you to stop the craziness of trying a new diet, losing the weight, gaining it back again, and then starting another diet.

My failure led me to more reading to try to determine why I was unsuccessful. This time I grabbed books that talked about our collective relationship with food. The books that influenced me the most were *The Omnivore's Dilemma* by Michael Pollan, *Mindless*

Eating by Brian Wansink, PhD, and *The End of Overeating* by David Kessler, MD. (See page 6 for some other helpful books—and even a movie—about our relationship with food.)

Each of them woke me up to ways that I could change my personal relationship with food. In *The Omnivore's Dilemma*, Michael Pollan traces the origins of a McDonald's meal to the cornfields and cattle feedlots. After reading this book, I realized that I knew almost nothing about where my food came from or what was in it. This wasn't just a problem for me to solve for myself, but one I knew I had better figure out if I was going to be a responsible parent.

I started reading the backs of food packages and I didn't like what I saw. For example, a Snapple that I purchased for my daughter had a label that read "All Natural" and ingredients that included high-fructose corn syrup and artificial colors. Huh? I was expecting the bottle to read "apple juice, pineapple juice, strawberry juice" since the front of the bottle had lovely photos of these fruits. Instead it had added sugar in the form of high-fructose corn syrup, the same stuff they use in Coca-Cola. That can't be right! Should I have just bought my two-year-old a Coke? Once I started digging into the nutrition facts of products, I began to realize that I had been duped over and over again. Being a good parent meant that I had to read the back of the label *before* I bought anything for my children. Then it became obvious that I had to start reading the labels for *my* food as well.

In *Mindless Eating*, Dr. Wansink describes an experiment: People are presented with a bowl of soup. They are not aware that as they eat, the bowl is constantly refilled via a tube at the bottom of the bowl. You would think that people would stop when they were full, right? Wrong. One guy, in twenty minutes, managed to eat four cups of soup! *Mindless Eating* is filled with similar stories about how we use our eyes instead of our stomachs to determine how much we should eat.

Without even thinking, I had been eating everything on my plate. Have you noticed how many fries they put on your plate at a restaurant? I was eating through a ton of fries without even noticing. Right after reading Wansink's book, I started to pay attention when I was eating fries and found that I actually wanted only a quarter of what was served to me. Or course, the easiest place to control portion size is at home. I bought a simple kitchen scale to get a handle on what I was consuming. I didn't use it punitively: "You can have only 4 ounces of steak," for example. Instead, I used it to figure out what 4 ounces of steak looked like so I could better judge how much I was really eating.

The last book that caught my attention was written by a former FDA commissioner under presidents Bush and Clinton, David A. Kessler. In *The End of Overeating*, Dr. Kessler outlines a large body of evidence that shows how fatty, salty, and sweet foods affect the same area of the brain as heroin. His theory is that food manufacturers (including restaurants and bakeries) have figured out what that perfect taste combination is and have increasingly used this information to make us buy more foods that have it.

Here are a few examples of the fatty, salty, and sweet food he is talking about:

Chicken, bacon, ranch pizza
Coffee Heath Bar Crunch ice cream
Oreo cookies
Buffalo chicken wings
Nacho Cheese Doritos

OUR RELATIONSHIP WITH FOOD

Fast Food Nation: The Dark Side of the American Meal by Eric Schlosser

Food Matters: A Guide to Conscious Eating with More Than 75 Recipes by Mark Bittman

In Defense of Food: An Eater's Manifesto by Michael Pollan

Food, Inc., a film by Robert Renner

My favorite example is a chocolate-covered caramel with salt sprinkled on the outside. I know exactly where to find these in the supermarket. Dr. Kessler would say that my brain got hardwired to love these because they hit a "bliss point" that made me crave them.

Do you notice how raw broccoli isn't on the list? The list is entirely processed food that someone created, most likely at a major food company.

This book freed me from guilt about my love of unhealthy foods. As I walked by the doughnut place around the corner from my house, I could now identify the powerful pull to grab a chocolate-glazed doughnut as my neurons fired and I tried to control my somewhat reasonable self. When I gave the urge a name—addiction—I was able to talk myself out of a doughnut most of the time.

The New, Healthier, Easier Path

Reading these books started me on a new type of journey. I quit the "I'm gonna lose 20 pounds in four weeks" trip and started the "I'm going to pay attention to what I eat and get healthier" concept.

Slowly, I learned how to deal with the enormous amount of food that surrounded me on a daily basis. I began to really see all the drive-throughs and large plates that cajoled me to eat more. And, I started to address the emotions that led me to eat when I wasn't hungry.

Did I try to give up meat, hike a mountain, and learn how to sauté perfect crisp-tender vegetables in one week? Heck, no. Life isn't a race—it is a journey. I was successful in losing weight because I changed how I ate and dealt with my food issues gradually. I am not offering you a diet plan that will save you from cupcakes forever. I'm quite sure you already know the areas of your diet that need fixing. If something isn't bugging you right now about your choices, then this is not the right book for you.

But if you do know what you want to fix, I'm your gal. I have found that multiple small changes to my diet have led to big results over time. For example, I started snacking on apples and peanut butter instead of cookies. From this simple change, I have more energy, I weigh less, and now I actually like apples and peanut butter *more* than cookies.

TOP 10 WAYS THIS BOOK WILL RESCUE YOU

1. **Eat for lasting weight loss.** Notice the cover of this book doesn't say, "Lose 15 pounds in two weeks!" Some books will help you lose 15 pounds in two weeks, but inevitably, you will put those 15 pounds back on, plus more. That's because you have deprived yourself of nutrition your body needs or of treats you feel you can't live without. So many times after not eating the foods we love, we end up binge eating them and gaining back the weight. Every sane source about weight loss says it is a "lifestyle" change and there is no time limit to your healthy eating and weight loss journey. Whatever amount of weight you want to lose, take the time to lose it right. It probably

took you years to add the pounds, and it may take you months, even years, to lose them. The good news is that those incremental changes add up to a healthier life and sustainable weight loss.

2. **Start tasting fresh food again.** Do you spend your money on Diet Coke? If so, your taste buds are getting slammed with an artificial sweetener that can prevent you from enjoying the flavor of a fresh strawberry, a crisp cucumber, or a tender green bean. Once you begin to taste the myriad of flavors fresh produce provides, you won't need as much cheese, butter, sugar, and salt for it to taste good. I am not suggesting that you will start to like unseasoned steamed veggies on salt-free brown rice. What I am hoping is that you will love sharing a whole pound of asparagus roasted with a mere tablespoon of olive oil (only 53 calories per serving and so yummy, page 196).

3. **Enjoy your food.** Life is too short to be constantly criticizing yourself for every morsel that crosses your lips. It is best to give in to your love of food and just indulge yourself when you come across something so delicious you can't resist it. Be proud of your choice to enjoy food.

4. **Make your favorite foods healthier.** We all know what meatloaf and mashed potatoes taste like. Is there a way to make them lighter without compromising their flavor? Sure! Is it hard? No! And your family might not even notice. Don't try to move from meatloaf to lentil loaf in one step. How about adding some mushrooms or more shredded veggies to your meatloaf (page 186)?

5. **Start with affordable, easy-to-find ingredients.** Why is there no sushi-grade tuna in this book? Because I can't find it at my regular grocery store. And even if I could find it, I probably couldn't afford it. There are enough healthy, affordable foods in our supermarkets to make the change to healthier eating. Just start in the produce section and fill your cart with colors. If you are lucky enough to live near a farmer's market, head there

for sparkling fresh produce. It's fun to shop for food where you know all the choices will be healthy and your food will taste incredible with very little effort on your part. Let the farmer do the work of creating healthy food whenever possible.

6. **Try new vegetables and whole grains.** I know it is intimidating to pick up and cook with ingredients that you have never tried before. I had that experience with parsnips. I didn't even know what a parsnip was until I met my husband. I found out they look like carrots, are a little sweeter, and taste great with mustard. Don't you want to be an example to your children and grandchildren? "Hey, look at Grannie, she eats kale for breakfast!" (Don't worry if you don't know how to cook kale—I didn't know either before I started Snack Girl.)

7. **Look for products with a short ingredient list.** I wish I could do it all, like Martha Stewart, but it ain't gonna happen. In a perfect world we'd all make our marinara sauce from scratch, but in the real world we often need or want an easier way. The good news is that major food manufacturers are listening to consumers who want fewer additives, preservatives, and sugar in their food, and there are new food products that are as close to homemade as you can get.

8. **Avoid anything artificial.** There is no reason to use artificial sweeteners, egg substitutes, or nonfat dairy if you are eating a healthy diet. You can lose weight without these products, and your food will taste better. Using only an egg white may be a great way to cut calories, but that means tossing away the nutrient-packed yolk. Where using the whole egg will help your food taste amazing, use it.

9. **Start giggling.** How do you make hard changes fun? By lightening up! No matter how depressed you are about the current state of your diet or the numbers on your scale, smile. Unless you live in a cave, every day you are surrounded by far more food than you could possibly eat. You drive by fast

food, walk by candy jars, and stop yourself from eating everything in sight—
All. Day. Long. It takes an iron will and a full night's sleep to pass by the free candy in the office. Begin to celebrate each time you walk past those candies without taking one. Next time you might not even notice them. Hopefully, this book will make you laugh about our collective dilemmas. A lot.

10. **Unstick your butt from the couch.** Yeah, that adhesive is *strong*. Take a few steps off the couch and that magnet will pull you right back down. My own butt was stuck for many years after having children. If you want to go sea kayaking with your honey, rock climbing with your best friend, or simply play more with your kids, try Snack Girl's five-minute plan and other doable suggestions for getting yourself unstuck.

If you act on the advice in this book, you will fill your shopping cart with the best food in the store without taking out a loan. When you push your cart up to the checkout lane, you will feel proud of what you have put in it. Your cart will be filled with fruits, vegetables, whole grains, and lean meats. You will be buying real food, and this shift will infuse your life with new energy. In addition, you will find inspiration for getting active without an expensive physical trainer or gym membership (unless you want one).

My goal is to teach you small steps that will ultimately rescue you from the danger of unhealthy food and eating habits. Maybe today, you will buy this book (one step). You may try one of my recipes, take a walk around the block, or buy a treadmill (three steps). You decide the steps that make sense to help you achieve lasting results.

Learn from this book, lose weight, eat well, get moving, and live a long, healthy life.

PART 1

Encouragement
and Guidance

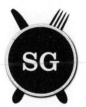

Healthy Weight and Healthy Image

I Have Tried _____ Diet and It Didn't Work!

Ever notice how everyone around you seems to be succeeding at losing weight and you're not? These people give you all this amazingly crazy advice: Give up all sugar! Start your day with a clove of fresh garlic! Juice all of your vegetables and never touch bacon again! Look at you, you need more vitamin D! Flush your colon!

Okay, maybe not "flush your colon."

If you have ever tried a diet, and most of us have, you know that it is incredibly challenging to radically change what you eat on a daily basis. For example, if you get up in the morning and pour yourself a bowl of Cheerios, it isn't going to be easy to start making steel-cut oatmeal that takes forty-five minutes to cook. You only have ten minutes before you need to be out the door!

So, if we can't cook, where do we eat? Walking distance from my office are pizza, bagels, more pizza, burgers, fries, and sandwiches. How many times a week do we just grab something nearby because we are too busy to do anything else?

Then, there is our baggage about food. You've been eating since the day you were born, and family, friends, coworkers, television, and billboards influence your relationship with food. Some of us have a full set of Samsonite when it comes to our eating habits. Our diets work for us until they stop working for us and we end up bigger and unhealthier than we should be.

There is good news. I believe that every time you tried a diet to lose weight you learned something about your relationship with food. You gleaned a valuable piece of information that showed you what you need to work on.

Several times a month, I receive an e-mail from a Snack Girl reader who wants to know what I think of different commercial weight loss solutions. The marketing for these products and plans is powerful. How many of us want to look like the "after" photo? We want to believe that what these companies are selling will solve our problem.

While I haven't tried all of them, I have checked them out for my readers. If you have tried any or all of these solutions, join the club! Hey, they seemed to have worked for someone, right?

Weight Loss Pills

I like to think of these as the "bad boys" of the diet world. They promise you instant success. All you have to do is give them your credit card number and the weight will just melt off. You will never be hungry again and you can just keep eating what you love.

Like a really cute guy or gal who tells you everything you want to hear, these plans are irresistible. But, just like that cute guy who probably isn't the man of your dreams, these pills leave a lot to be desired. Most of the time, people find that the pills don't work as promised. Of all the over-the-counter diet quick fixes, only one, Alli, has been approved by the FDA (as of 2012). Alli's side effects include frequent or hard-to-control bowel movements and there is a slight chance of serious liver injury. Sound like fun?

In the "nondrug" corner are the over-the-counter supplements such as Hoodia, Green Tea Extract, Hydroxycut, and Estrin-D, among others. These pills can make claims about their efficacy without any scientific evidence because they are in the "supplement" category. (Why the FDA doesn't monitor claims from supplements is a mystery to me.) Many of these diet pills contain caffeine and have side effects such as dizziness, insomnia, and nausea.

Just for fun, let's say that scientists did create a weight loss pill that made the pounds melt off. This is such a hot area of drug company research it could happen one day. Would that solve your problem?

Probably not.

Why? Let me give you an example. There is a group of amazing drugs that help people who suffer with depression, anxiety, post-traumatic stress disorder, and other emotional issues. These drugs, which include Prozac, Xanax, and Zoloft, make a difference for millions of people.

I am one of those people. I suffer from anxiety and have been prescribed a drug called Lorazepam (Ativan). This little pill wipes away all my tension and helps me to sleep when I am gripping my bed sheets with anxiety. The sad part is that it doesn't solve the problem that is keeping me up at night and it comes with a serious side effect.

The last time I asked for a refill for my prescription my doctor said she would give it to me only if I started walking. She wasn't going to give me any more of my beloved drug unless I got out of my office chair and got outside for a few minutes a day.

So which do you think works better for me: Lorazepam or walking? Walking! Surprised? I find that if I get a walk in, I don't wake up worried in the middle of the night. Before walking regularly, I used to think relaxing was sitting on the couch, or drinking a glass of wine. Yes, I knew that exercise made me feel good but I didn't associate it with becoming calmer.

It turns out that walking outside helps me unwind better than watching television, reading, or sitting inside alone for a few minutes. Looking up at the sky, smelling the fresh air, breathing deep breaths, all combine to give me a feeling of peace. The side effects of walking have been that my waist has slimmed down a couple of inches, my cholesterol levels are lower, and I can (mostly) keep up with my children.

Is walking harder than taking a pill? Of course! Sometimes you have to work at things to make change happen.

Lesson from Diet Pills

Taking a diet pill will not fix where you have gotten yourself after months or years of overeating. Even if it does work, like the Lorazepam for my anxiety, it isn't a long-term solution. Everyone I know who has gotten healthy and lost weight has had to learn how to make better food choices, cook, and get more exercise. Don't feel bad if you don't cook or work out; you have time to change that! I hope to convince you that the side effects of these new activities will be much more pleasant than nausea, diarrhea, and dizziness.

Prepackaged Food, Diet Shakes, Cleanses, and Juice Fasts

If you watch any daytime television, you have heard the ad, "Just a shake for breakfast, another for lunch, and a reasonable dinner and you could be a hundred pounds lighter, just like me." I like to think of these diets as extreme diet makeovers. All you have to do is stop eating everything that you usually eat and you will lose weight.

I don't know about you, but I would be seriously hungry all day with just a beverage for breakfast and lunch. My role in the morning is to make my children breakfast and pack their lunch. What kind of example am I setting by drinking my breakfast from a can? I know my kids would be demanding that shake if they saw me drink it. If I attempted one of these diets, I would have to wait until they left and then drink my breakfast. I can't imagine hiding my diet shake habit from my children.

On the other hand, it does seem to be an easy choice. You write a hefty check, order meals, maybe you get a counselor, and then just follow their plan.

But how is this different from the magical diet pills?

The good news is that you are following a nutrition plan that has some thought put into it, but are you really making the shift to a healthier lifestyle? You outsourced all the work to a company, and now you're simply just following the numbers. A lack of nutritional knowledge as well as an understanding of what your body needs led you to try the program. Can you buy meals and drink shakes and lose weight? Absolutely. Will you still have to learn how to cook something to become healthy? Yes.

These plans also seem really impractical if you want to celebrate a wedding anniversary or a best friend's birthday. I *love* my treats and I think it is best to learn how to incorporate them into your healthy lifestyle while you are losing weight.

How about a cleanse to help you lose weight? I love the idea that we can clean our insides as well as our outsides. For example, the Lemon Detox diet has you drink six to eight glasses per day of a mixture of lemon juice, maple syrup, a wee bit of cayenne pepper, and water. After seven to ten days you will be clean! I would guess that you would also be hankering for a bacon cheeseburger.

Juice fasts are another type of cleansing diet. In a 2010 documentary called *Fat, Sick, and Nearly Dead*, Joe Cross, a 300-pound Australian man with an autoimmune disease, decides to drive across America, juicer in tow. He goes on a sixty-day juice fast, drinking only the juices from fruits and vegetables, and loses 80 pounds. This guy is cute, so the "before" and "after" photos are quite dramatic. He goes from teddy bear to *hot*.

> **TOP DIETS FEATURING PREPACKAGED MEALS AND SHAKES**
>
> Jenny Craig
>
> MediFast
>
> Slim-Fast
>
> Nutrisystem

Mr. Hot Guy was actually at my local Whole Foods hawking $400 juicers. But I don't have the space or the dough for a juicer, and won't I be really hungry if all I consume is juice?

My first problem with a liquid cleanse or juice fast is how impractical it would be. Most days, I prepare breakfast, lunch, and dinner for my family. How am I supposed to not eat? I have enough trouble with the candy bowl at work or the Dunkin' Donuts drive-through that I pass every day. I know I don't have the willpower to not eat when lovely food is in front of me and I am starving.

Also, when you eat less, your metabolism slows down to conserve energy. You will burn some fat, but then your body kicks down a notch to keep you alive until the next meal. Not getting enough nutrients during fasting diets can lead to symptoms such as fatigue, dizziness, constipation, and dehydration. Sound familiar?

Lesson from Prepackaged Meals, Diet Shakes, Cleanses, and Juice Fasts

The concept that you must replace what you are eating with something else is a good one. Yes, if you are trying to change your diet, you need to take a good hard look at what you are eating and make adjustments. But you don't need to buy prepackaged food, diet shakes, or an expensive juicer to make the shift to a thinner, healthier you.

TOP "BOGEYMAN" DIETS

The South Beach Diet
by Arthur Agatston, MD

The Zone Diet
by Barry Sears, PhD

The Dukan Diet
by Pierre Dukan, MD

The Atkins Diet
by Robert Atkins, MD

Eat to Live
by Joel Fuhrman, MD

Forks Over Knives
edited by Gene Stone

The Diet "Bogeyman" Approach

Something is hiding in your food, and it is *making you fat!* These diets are the ones that scare you with their intensity, grab headlines in the newspapers, and sell a lot of books because they are so simple. Their writers are usually doctors and they find that a specific macronutrient, like protein, carbohydrates, fat, or a specific vitamin or mineral, like vitamin D, is the key to weight loss. These diets seem to have many scientific studies supporting their thesis and a beautiful spokesperson who has lost a lot of weight using their plan.

For example, there is the Atkins Diet created by Dr. Robert Atkins. His research led him to the conclusion that carbohydrates are the key to weight loss. Eat more protein (including his protein bars) and less bread, rice, starchy vegetables, baked goods, and fruit and you are on your way to thin. This approach leaves you with a lot of meat, fish, and poultry to eat, which contain zero carbohydrates.

In direct contrast to the Atkins Diet, we have *Eat to Live* by Joel Fuhrman, MD. It proclaims that you will lose 20 pounds or more in six weeks. Hooray! During those six weeks you get to give up animal and dairy products, between-meal snacks, oils, and fruit juice. His recommendation is to stick to plant-based foods to reduce your weight and your risk of disease.

Argh! Can't they make up their minds?

If you have tried either of these, and I have, you might find yourself constipated and longing for a salad, or bloated and longing for a steak. Will either approach solve your weight loss problem? I don't know. My conclusion is that either approach is far too extreme for my life. Maybe if I were living alone and in control of my entire daily food intake and could cook only what I wanted to eat, I could give up carbohydrates or all animal products. Most of us aren't in this position.

The nice thing about these diets is that there is usually some wisdom in them, and often there is scientific research supporting their theories about how to lose weight. Yes, if you eat less meat and saturated fat, you will get healthier. Yes, if you eat fewer highly processed carbohydrates (think: white bread, Oreos, Fritos) and more protein, you will be less hungry and lose pounds.

But many people (including me) buy these books, only to have them end up at our garage sales. Why? Most of us give these diets a good try for a few days or weeks and then give up. Then we buy another book that looks like it has the key to success, try it, and give it to our brother when we can't make the new plan work for us.

You really feel like a failure when you can't stick to these diets because they seem so easy, but the truth is that they are too rigid for most of us to maintain. These are also the trendy diets that everyone is trying and talking about at the same time, and it may seem that they're working for everyone but you. You can feel really lousy when you fail at them. But check back with your friends after six months and see how they're doing.

Lesson from Bogeyman Diets

You can make adjustments in your macronutrient levels and lose weight, but if the plan isn't sustainable for you, you won't keep weight off in the long term. Don't worry, at least you learned (for example) that more protein helped you stay full or eating fewer empty carbohydrates gave you energy. Take all the information you can get from these plans to make informed decisions about your diet. If you eliminate a specific type of food from your diet, you learn something about your body. It is like you did a little scientific experiment on yourself. How fun!

For example, I spent the entire day at a yoga retreat center where all the food was vegan and no sugar was added to any of the dishes. I got there at 6 a.m. and at about 3 p.m., I started to crave something sweet. I was there to learn how to reduce my level of anxiety and I found myself starting to lose it because of my lust for a cookie.

What did I do?

Like all the other yogis, I had a candy stash in my car. I ran out when no one was looking and grabbed a handful of malted milk balls. Problem solved. Clearly I needed sugar a wee bit more than I thought I did.

Online Food Journaling Tools and Weight Watchers

Now, we get to the good stuff! Instead of someone else defining your weight loss goals, you take control. Write down everything you eat using a notebook or the Internet (or both). This tool, called food journaling, leads to success because people become aware of exactly what and how much they eat every day.

You can set a calorie goal and total up the numbers at the end of the day. Weight Watchers assigns "PointsPlus" values to food and you aim to eat close to the PointsPlus total you are allotted.

If you use an online tool, such as MyFitnessPal.com, or join WeightWatchers .com you can participate in the community aspect of the program. It can be super fun to become part of a group of people who have the same goals and challenges that you have.

I know people who lost weight and kept it off because they started keeping a food journal. They just didn't realize that they ate a cookie, a doughnut, *and* a bowl of ice cream all in one day. By recording everything they ate they could see where those extra calories (and pounds) were coming from, and make mindful decisions about what they really wanted to eat.

The Weight Watchers program in 2012 takes calorie counting one step further and tries to help you to decide what to eat. The diet emphasizes eating fruits and vegetables to help people feel full on the same amount of food that they usually eat, but with fewer calories. In fact, on this program, you don't even count fruits and nonstarchy vegetables as part of your daily calorie goal. I love the emphasis on eating fruits and vegetables because I think it is a win-win. What health professional isn't telling us to eat more fruits and vegetables? In 2009, the Centers for Disease Control reported that only 26 percent of adults in the United States were eating three or more vegetables per day. What is the other 74 percent eating?

Weight Watchers is based on solid research that indicates that you can eat the same *volume* of food and feel full, but eat fewer calories and lose weight. Picture a plate with a large steak, a pile of potatoes, and a few green beans. See that? Now picture the plate with 3 ounces of steak, a small potato, and salad covering the rest of the plate. Guess what? You can feel full with the second plate and lose weight. Many of the recipes on Snack-Girl.com and in this book are focused on increasing the volume of fruits and vegetables in your diet.

My big problem with food journaling and Weight Watchers was that I would get to the end of my day and realize that I couldn't have that beer, ice cream, or pizza and stay within my limit. My willpower was not strong enough to stop me from going over my limit and then I would feel guilty (which led to more eating).

Lesson from Food Journaling and Weight Watchers

I think everyone should try food journaling for at least one day. Keep a small pad or notebook and pen (or your smartphone or tablet if you're so inclined) with you and write down a list of everything—and I mean everything—you eat. I like to note the time of day and how I was feeling at the time. For example:

7:00 a.m.	Scrambled eggs, coffee. Half my son's leftover buttered English muffin—Rushed
10:00 a.m.	Apple, hard-boiled egg—Hungry
12:30 p.m	Ham sandwich, banana, cookie—Sleepy
3:00 p.m.	Coffee, four Hershey's Kisses—Bored
6:00 p.m.	Beef chili, salad, rice, beer—Hungry
10:00 p.m.	Potato Chips—Horny

You will begin to notice patterns to your eating that have nothing to do with being hungry and *that*, my dear reader, is where you start. You can lose a lot of weight if you stop eating when you aren't hungry.

Don't forget to take a hard look at what you are drinking. Soda, juice, and alcohol all have empty calories that could be sneaking up on you. If you cut out just one 12-ounce sugary soda per day, you will save 1,400 calories over ten days. This type of small step can lead to a big difference in your waistline.

Diet Plan Lessons

I may have failed at every diet I tried, but I learned something from each experience. I took the information I gathered and I tried to stop beating myself up. I adopted a new saying that would keep me going when I felt discouraged:

Begin again

Sounds like something written on a groovy tea bag, doesn't it? Begin again—not "start again," because that would mean I was at the beginning of the journey. Not "try again" because that would mean I had failed.

Begin again!

How did I begin again? I kept looking for new simple, small steps that worked. I started to feel good about my growing knowledge of what worked and stopped worrying about what didn't. Hey, it's a process!

I Hate Looking at Myself in the Mirror

When you look in the mirror, what do you see? Do you look at the sparkle in your eyes or the chub around your middle? I've thought a lot about a soft middle because I have one. My eyes are drawn to it whenever I pass a reflective surface. Guess what? Nobody cares about my middle except me. I've asked my husband a bunch of times, "Do you wish I were less round?" and he looks at me as if I'm nuts.

Here's an experiment for you. The next time you go to the salon or barbershop, start reading *People, Cosmopolitan,* or *Men's Health* or whatever other glossy magazine with photos of people that may be lying around. Look down at the photos and then look up at all the people sitting in the room. Does anyone there actually look like any of the photos in the magazine? If you want to stare, just put on some dark glasses. Unless you happen to be in a salon where they service models, my guess is that no one looks anything like those photos, including you.

I hear a lot from Snack Girl readers about those "last 10 pounds." Are those the 10 pounds that will magically turn them into a magazine-ready version of themselves? I wonder, Is this a real health issue, or a body image issue? Are these readers comparing their bodies to images that are unattainable and hoping if they just give up that last daily glass of wine, they'll get there? We all do it, including me. But why do we torture ourselves?

My feminist mother raised me to believe that I had to rely on my brains to create a successful life. She never put a dollop of makeup on my face and hardly ever put any on her own. I dodged the teenage years of experimenting with beauty products, fashion, and hairstyles because I was a nerdy jock. I thought I was immune to the magazines, billboards, and television shows with their "perfect" starlets. I didn't need to be beautiful because I was smart. You can just imagine how empowered I felt.

Once when I was in my late twenties, visiting my parents in Los Angeles, my mother decided that I needed a great haircut and graciously gave me a present of an appointment at a Beverly Hills salon. The stylist was famous for cutting the hair of a number of stars, Renée Zellweger among them.

When I walked in the door I saw an extraordinarily beautiful group of women (just like they had stepped out of a magazine!). They had perfect teeth, hair, and nails and their bodies seemed to range from size 0 to 2.

My size 12 self had never felt more hideous. I literally felt like hiding under my chair as I read my *People*.

A very handsome guy took me to a basin to wash my hair. I felt so uncomfortable that I said, "I feel so ugly!!"

He stopped massaging my head, looked down at me, and said, "You are the most beautiful woman in this room. You have soft round curves and you have a great smile on your face. These women take laxatives and diet pills to achieve their ideal weight, which turns them into shrews. I would much rather go out with you than any of them."

And now he is my husband. (Just kidding!)

I had internalized our cultural definition of beauty and decided that I was ugly because I didn't fit it. This lovely man woke me up! In his opinion, trying to be picture perfect made the outwardly stunning women too grumpy to be attractive (which is really funny when you think about it).

Whatever your weight loss goal, start accepting yourself—*now*. Nobody is comparing you to Angelina Jolie, Tom Cruise, or Halle Berry. Their images stare at us from every supermarket checkout counter—but they don't define beauty.

You get to define beauty.

If you find yourself staring at your muffin top when you look in the mirror, look up. Look at your face and decide that it is a waste of time to obsess over imperfections that do not encompass or define who you are. I've never met one person whose entire self was constructed around a muffin top.

Yes, okay, I know you don't think it is attractive, but I would bet there is much about you that is more beautiful than you think.

Healthy Versus Skinny

When did "skinny" get to be such an important word in our lexicon? Skinny bitch, skinny margaritas, skinny jeans. Sheesh. I remember when "skinny" meant that you looked like you needed to eat something.

In my opinion "skinny" shouldn't be a positive lifestyle choice. The Merriam-Webster dictionary definition of the word "skinny" is: *Lacking sufficient flesh: very thin; emaciated.*

Other words that come to mind: gaunt, scrawny, haggard.

Do any of these words make you think "healthy"? They make me think of Gandhi on a hunger strike.

It is important to realize that your body shape may be different from society's vision of thin and still be healthy.

Body Mass Index (BMI)

How do you assess what is a healthy weight for you? Many books and doctors will point you to the Body Mass Index as the definitive way to calculate your healthy weight.

BMI uses your height and weight to calculate a number that indicates if you are underweight, normal, overweight, or obese. It is a very simple measure that can completely miss its mark.

When I was twenty-eight, I was introduced to BMI at a routine physical. The nurse practitioner was looking down at a sheet of paper when she pronounced that I was overweight. I was shocked because at the time I was swimming a hundred laps per day, five times a week. My stomach was flat (the kind of flat I will never see again after giving birth to two children). I fit well in my clothes and I felt like I could climb Mount Everest. I was in killer shape. But, I was 5 feet 6 inches tall and weighed 165 pounds and that, my friends, put me in the "overweight" category of the BMI.

I looked straight at the nurse and said, "Take a good look at me. Tell me again that I am overweight." She looked at me and reinforced the BMI finding, which I found very strange.

Turns out that I'm not the only one having strange conversations with health practitioners about BMI. Brad Pitt, Kobe Bryant, and George Clooney are also overweight if you look at their BMI (their height and weight information can be found on celebrity websites). I wish I could be a fly on the wall for those checkups!

The problem with BMI is that it doesn't differentiate between weight from fat and weight from bone and muscle. Because bone is denser than muscle and muscle is twice as dense as fat, you could be considered overweight because you have strong bones and good muscle tone for your height, a combination that makes you heavier than average.

What is important is what percentage of your body is made up of fat. You could have a "normal" BMI and still have too much fat to be healthy.

What else could you use to help determine your healthy weight? Researchers are talking about waist circumference as a great way to measure abdominal fat. My grandmother could have told them that. The old commercials for Special K cereal have this wisdom embedded. Does anyone else remember, "Can you pinch more than an inch?" It turns out that waist-to-height ratios are better at predicting diabetes, hypertension, and cardiovascular disease than BMI.

Toss out your scale and go find yourself a tape measure. Next you need to find your waist. Get naked in front of a mirror and locate the top of your hipbone. Place the tape measure evenly around the abdomen at this level. Measure the circumference; be sure to relax (don't suck in your stomach) and don't pull the tape too tight.

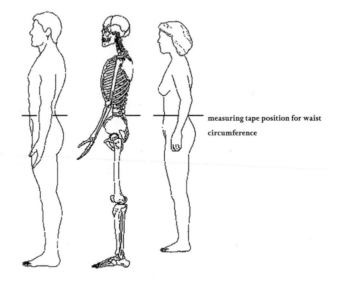

measuring tape position for waist circumference

Now that you have a baseline measurement, what does it mean? Again, you have to realize that the suggestion for a healthy waist circumference is an average over the population, and scientific studies are ongoing to determine the ideal measure. In 2012, the National Institutes of Health stated that the risk of heart disease and type 2 diabetes increases when waist size is greater than 35 inches for women and 40 inches for men.

Here is another example of why a tape measure is a better way to assess your health than a scale. Let's say you have a small pudge and you want to get rid of it. You could conceivably gain weight by adding muscle (via weight training) and look slimmer.

I like to use a tape measure around my waist to determine if I have been hitting the wine and cheese too much. Or I use my favorite pair of jeans. The waist of my jeans falls naturally at the top of my hipbone. Too tight? I lay off the Cheddar and Cabernet for a couple of days.

Physicals and Healthy Habits

What other measures could you use to determine if you are healthy? A physical provides all sorts of test results.

I never went for a physical until I had children, but now that I want to meet my grandchildren I make it a priority. The urinalysis, blood pressure, and blood glucose tests and pelvic and breast exams could help you catch a potential problem before it is too late to do something about it. Once your doctor gives you the results, you can decide what to do with the information.

If we are lucky, our doctors have the same health philosophy as we do and help us achieve our goals. Unfortunately, too often, our doctors don't have the time (and most don't have the training) to help us plan a strategy when it comes to diet. For example, when my doctor told me to lose weight, he didn't really explain how to do it. He had to move on to his next patient.

Healthy is not about being skinny or thin. It is choosing to do the obvious—all those things that years of research have been screaming at us to do. Eat fruits, vegetables, whole grains, fish/lean meats—and treats in moderation. Get enough exercise and sleep. Don't drink yourself into a stupor every night with a bag of chips in front of the television. These habits are obvious but for many—myself included—tough to accomplish. Good health is not about perfection; it's about moving slowly and steadily toward a long-term goal.

Healthy Cooking

All I Can Cook Is Hamburgers and I Should Be Eating Vegetables

What was the first dish you ever learned to cook? I bet if anyone showed you how to use the stove when you were a child they taught you how to scramble eggs. There is something magical about watching the liquid egg turn into solid yellow sunshine. Did they take the time to teach you anything else?

Way back in 1996, a survey revealed that 53 percent of Americans feel they have less knowledge and fewer cooking skills than their mothers and grandmothers (they forget the fathers, I guess). Another survey in 2011 reported that 28 percent of Americans don't know how to cook. If almost a third of the country isn't cooking regularly, who is buying all that stuff at Williams-Sonoma? Do people just hang all those shiny pans in their kitchens for show?

I am not in the 28 percent of noncooks because my dad turned me into his sous-chef at an early age. I didn't know what a sous-chef (sounds like "sue chef") was for the longest time, until I took seventh-grade French. Basically, a sous-chef is a person who preps all the ingredients for the main chef. My dad had me chopping onions and celery, opening cans of tomatoes, and mincing garlic as soon as I could use a knife without hurting myself. Unfortunately, he didn't get around to showing me how to hold my knife properly. My knife skills didn't mature until I was forty-three, and my emotional maturity is still questionable.

I spent a lot of time hiding whenever I heard the call for the "sue chef" because I wanted to do something else, like talking on the phone with my friends, examining the cracks on the ceiling, or watching grass grow. Chopping was such a pain!

I had other food responsibilities in addition to my chef duties. When I learned how to drive, I did the grocery shopping for my family every week. This was considered payback for the car that they let me use, a dirty penny–colored Volkswagen Rabbit, as well as the exorbitant cost of insuring a teenage driver in the suburbs of New York City. My dad would give me a list and then I would have to fight for a parking space at the grocery store, spend an hour trying to find all the gourmet ingredients he wanted, and stand in line for twenty minutes as people fumbled for their checkbooks. I absolutely hated it.

Then, there was the cleaning. After dinner, my mother, sister, and I had to clean up the hurricane of mess left all over the kitchen after my dad finished cooking. He made sure he had all the fun and left all the hard work to the rest of us. I resented the time I spent washing up after the chef. This predisposed me to hate being in the kitchen and to despise washing pots.

The positive aspect of my father's cooking is that he made great food from wonderful cookbooks, including Julia Child's *Mastering the Art of French Cooking* and (my personal favorite) Marcella Hazan's *Essentials of Classic Italian Cooking*. We ate gourmet meals most nights of the week, but I wasn't grateful.

When I left for college, I was thrilled not to have to be anyone's chef, maid, or shopper and I signed up for the dining hall's meal plan. I was in heaven for about two weeks until I realized that all they were going to serve was hamburgers, fries, chicken nuggets, and pizza for the whole semester. I found that I couldn't eat because I was so used to home-cooked food made with fresh ingredients. My stomach began to hurt and I started to dread eating at the dining hall.

Fortunately, my dormitory had rooms with efficiency kitchens and I managed to switch into one of these as soon as I could. Now, I had to figure out how to cook.

When my doctor discovered I was anemic, she asked me what I was eating. I answered, "Macaroni and cheese, ramen noodles, and pizza. But I add peas to the macaroni and cheese and ramen noodles to get some vegetables." She frowned and told me to start eating healthier but didn't explain how to go about it. I was too busy putting myself through college, working part-time and studying full-time, to implement any real changes. I didn't have much money and I felt that I didn't have the time to cook real food, even though I knew what it was.

Even if I had known how to cook, I had another problem: I was living in a food desert in Brooklyn, New York. The closest grocery store was a fifteen-minute walk, it was expensive, and it smelled strongly of ammonia. This store was grimy and the fresh vegetables looked a bit, well, aged. It took me a year to figure out I had to take the subway to Chinatown to get fresh vegetables and fruit for a reasonable price. So much for not being a shopper anymore!

It wasn't until I went off to graduate school that I started to learn how to cook for myself. I subscribed to *Gourmet* (only $12 a year) and began to experiment in the kitchen and feed my friends for fun. I spent some time burning stuff and turning out borderline-edible meals. Every once in a while, I would make something truly delicious and use my scissors to cut the recipe out of the magazine. After five years, I had about fifteen recipes that I enjoyed making.

In two ways, I was lucky. I had been introduced to well-made, fresh food at a young age, and I had time in graduate school to experiment in the kitchen. Did I ever love to cook? *No.* Do I love to cook now? *No.* Am I ever going to love cooking? Some days I love it, because it can feel like a satisfying accomplishment when I manage to turn out an enjoyable meal that nourishes my family.

The first thing you have to do to become a healthy cook is admit that cooking is a skill that takes practice, and you may never *want* to do it. The problem is that the route to healthy includes preparing your own meals from fresh ingredients. You cannot just eat McDonald's salads or Subway subs (I don't care what Jared says) and be healthy.

Once you start mastering some basic skills, you will find out that *your* food tastes better than anything you have purchased at a fast-food venue. Trust me, it may take a while, but you will have an epiphany about how crappy the food is at many restaurants when you start to get a handle on cooking.

Get Thee Some Vegetables!

Most of us can put together a salad without much help. I have a pal who lived as a street musician for a while. He and his friends used to make salad in a plastic bag— toss in the lettuce and some dressing, shake it up, and eat it with their hands. Hey, it isn't fancy but these were some healthy musicians. I'm not suggesting you try this if you live in your own home and have things like bowls and silverware, but I do think it is interesting what kind of meals you can create with very little preparation.

If you are like me, you arrive at the grocery store having already figured out the easy part of the equation. Sure, you can always roast some chicken, grill a steak, or put together a meatloaf. The hard part is when you are standing there in the produce section and all these vegetables are looking at you. Actually, only the potatoes are looking at you because they have eyes (sorry, I spend a lot of time with a six-year-old). When I peek into other people's carts in my grocery store, I am always amazed at how few fresh vegetables are being taken to the checkout counter. (Walk around your store with mirrored sunglasses and you can do a lot of spying.)

After doing my research about dieting, it became clear that one thing I could do to lose weight and get healthier was fill half my plate with vegetables. Have you seen the MyPlate icon from the USDA? Protein takes up only a quarter of the plate; the rest is filled with vegetables, whole grains, and fruits. It is the opposite of most of our plates, heaped with our big slabs of meat, piles of potatoes, and a little sad side of vegetables. When I fill half my plate with vegetables, my body seems to run better and I have more energy. I don't get that overstuffed feeling that happens when you eat too much high-calorie food. It's worth a try, isn't it? But you do have to cook some vegetables.

Using a Knife

The first painful fact about vegetables is that you will have to peel, slice, chop, dice, or shred them if they are to cook in a reasonable amount of time. I know that when I'm tired the last thing I want to do is get out my knife and cutting board, but I find whacking a broccoli crown into pieces is an excellent way to get out the frustrations at the end of the day. To tame the savage beasts that are baying at the kitchen counter (aka my hungry children, impatient for dinner), I start handing out fresh carrot or celery sticks, or slices of red pepper. Frequently, my children will demand ranch dressing for a dip, everybody starts munching, and that buys me time to cook.

The first step on your cooking journey is buying a good, sharp knife. You need only one knife, called a "chef's knife," for most tasks in the kitchen. Get an 8- or 10-inch knife; it may seem big at first, but a sharp, heavy knife will do most of the work of slicing and dicing for you. My chef's knife and cutting board are the most utilized tools in my kitchen.

If you want to do some research before you buy, subscribe to the *Consumer Reports* website to look at options and price points, or just go to your local gourmet store (I did my hands-on research at Williams-Sonoma). The Reluctant Gourmet (reluctantgourmet.com) is another great resource for the beginning cook. He explains all the tools and ways to choose the best one for you.

Now that you have your knife, you must learn how to use it. I put a great video on Snack Girl (www.snack-girl.com/snack/how-chop-vegetables/) on how to hold a knife. YouTube is also a fantastic resource for learning knife skills. (Or any how-to you are confused about. I once unclogged a sink with my iPod playing a video in one hand and my plunger in the other.)

If you have the time and money, consider taking a class at your local cooking school or store. I did this and found that having an instructor correct me about a million times got me controlling my knife to the point that I could work in a professional kitchen (in my dreams). I did begin to understand how one could enjoy chopping and I was proud of my new skills.

Once you get a sharp knife, learn how to use it, and start practicing on some willing vegetables, you will have jumped over one of the biggest hurdles to learning how to cook efficiently. You might even start enjoying it. Fingers crossed (and hopefully not bandaged).

Is This Going to Cost Me?

Alice Waters, an activist chef and major proponent of organic food, famously defended paying $4 per pound for organic grapes when she appeared on *60 Minutes*, proclaiming:

> **We make decisions every day about what we are going to eat. And some people want to buy Nike shoes: two pairs! And other people want to eat [organic] grapes and nourish themselves. I pay a little extra but this is what I want to do.**

I am a huge fan of Alice Waters, but I cringed because I know that there are plenty of people who can't afford those grapes or the new Nike shoes.

For those of us who work with a "Payless Nike knock-off" budget, we need food solutions that we can afford. The fact is that if you look at price per calorie, processed food can't be beat. A package of cookies at my local dollar store has 2,000 calories and costs, you guessed it, one dollar. If I am lucky, for one dollar I can get two apples for 160 calories of nutritious food. The good news is that most of us need *fewer* calories, so choosing healthier food is easy.

What are the most affordable healthy foods? According to the 2013 EatingWell .com article, "12 Superfoods to Help You Eat Healthy for $1 or Less," the cheapest healthy foods are lentils, oats, kale, almonds, tea, oranges, canned tuna, peanut butter, apples, eggs, carrots, and cabbage. The article stipulates that "cheap" means $1 or less *per serving*, so don't get too excited. What is true is that you can find all of these foods year round in your supermarket and they are both healthy and affordable. The recipe section in the second half of the book uses almost all of these ingredients and many more that aren't on the list, such as dried kidney beans, onions, potatoes, and frozen corn.

Organic? Local? Supermarket?

When I was a kid, we bought our vegetables at either the grocery store or, in the summer, the local farm stand. Now I have a choice between my Stop & Shop, Whole Food's mostly organic produce, farm stands, farmer's markets (both winter and summer), and a farm share. Also called a CSA (community-supported agriculture), a farm share is when you pay for an entire season of produce from a local farm upfront and receive whatever produce they have picked every week.

There have been times in my life where I strolled through a farmer's market happily buying $6 per pound peaches because I was loaded with money and time. Other times in my life (post children), I have been happy to find peaches for $1.50 per pound in my supermarket as I sprint through the store. Do I feel bad that I stopped being able to afford organic, locally farmed produce? Honestly, I am just happy that I can afford fresh fruits and vegetables.

If you have the time to visit your local farmer's market and stock up on the freshest seasonal produce, it can be an incredibly rewarding experience. You are outdoors, maybe you run into a friend or neighbor, and you get to know the people who grow your food. The increase in the number of these markets around the country is a testament to how fun and rewarding they are to have in your community. Organic produce is better for the environment, but it can be expensive, and depending on where you live, may not be easy to find. I did a comparison between Whole Foods and my Stop & Shop and found if I had bought all organic products and produce at Whole Foods, I would have spent twice as much for the same amount of conventional food at Stop & Shop.

For those of you who are overwhelmed by the non-GMO, local, organic, and fair trade produce, just stop worrying about it. If your cart looks like a rainbow of fruits and vegetables, you have made a choice to support your health.

That rainbow should include the fruits and vegetables in the "Dirty Dozen," a list of the twelve foods most contaminated by pesticide residue compiled every year by the Environmental Working Group (EWG). EWG is a nonprofit environmental organization formed "to use the power of public information to protect public health and the environment." Their Dirty Dozen list is scary because it includes many of the foods some of us eat every day. In 2012, apples were first on the list, followed by celery (find the full list at ewg.org). It is, of course, important for groups other than the government to watch over our health. The problem is that the EWG is promoting the idea that this produce is "dirty." Is the apple that you pick up at the supermarket filthy with pesticides? A specific apple may have been treated with pesticide, and, yes, there may be residue on (or in) the apple. But is that residue harmful to you?

The president and founder of EWG, Ken Cook, stated in 2010,

We recommend that people eat healthy by eating more fruits and vegetables, whether conventional or organic . . . The health benefits of a diet rich in fruits and vegetables outweigh the risks of pesticide exposure.

The Dirty Dozen is about *how many* different pesticides are found on a given type of produce. For example, in 2012, celery tested positive for 57 different pesticides. This result does not mean there are 57 pesticides on one bunch of celery but that the farmers throughout the country and world use 57 different pesticides that remain on celery when it gets to the supermarket. EWG is not saying that the *amount* of pesticide on the bunch of celery you hold in your hand is dangerous to your health. What they are saying is that you can lower your pesticide residue intake by avoiding the twelve most contaminated fruits and vegetables. Minimizing pesticide exposure may be important to you, but it should not stop you from eating a healthy array of produce.

The Produce Section

So here you are in the produce section, and how are you going to get some good stuff? First, take a look at the prices. Produce that is in season is much less expensive than produce that is grown in greenhouses. For example, asparagus is a spring vegetable. In October, I found asparagus from South America that sold for $3 per pound. In January, asparagus was $6 per pound (ouch). Obviously, October is spring in South America so we get a bunch of fresh asparagus. January is not spring anywhere, so this is probably coming from more expensive greenhouse growers. So, I buy asparagus in October and March through May (when the U.S. crop starts to show up in my supermarket).

You don't have to spend a lot of time learning the seasons of fruits and vegetables. What I do is look for the sale signs and then, if I have time, I quiz the produce manager. "When did you get this? Why is it on sale?" Most big grocery stores have a manager who knows where they get their produce, when it is coming in, and what determines the price. I'm amazed at how much I have learned just by harassing these men and women. If you're shy, check out Produce Geek (www.producegeek.com) for weekly posts on what you will find in the sale aisles of your grocery store. In December, for example, Produce Geek will alert you to the blueberries rolling into the store (not literally) because it is the beginning of the summer in Chile. Hooray! Blueberries for Christmas!

After you see if there are any good deals, you need to closely examine the produce to ensure it is fresh. Pick it up, smell it, examine it for bruises, and buy only the best stuff. I don't care if your recipe calls for cauliflower. If the cauliflower has mushy brown patches, don't buy it. Don't be afraid to swap in broccoli if the broccoli looks better. If your vegetables aren't good before you cook them, they won't taste good after they're cooked.

If you can't afford fresh produce, don't give up on eating vegetables. Frozen vegetables are a great option because they are picked and processed at the peak of freshness. In fact, some frozen produce can have more nutrients than fresh, because fresh produce starts to lose nutrients soon after it is picked. The other nice thing about frozen produce is that you don't have to get out your knife and cutting board. Many of the recipes in this book use frozen produce because it is easy, cheap, and nonperishable— you don't have to worry that it will go bad if you don't cook it right away.

Cooking Vegetables the Easy Way

Now that you have your beautiful produce and chef's knife, you can start cooking. I was raised with boiled vegetables that lacked flavor, texture, and sometimes smelled like rotten eggs. Yuck! It wasn't until I went on the second date with an Australian guy, who became my husband, that I got a clue about vegetables. Were his vegetable skills important in our fledgling relationship? Let's just say the guy knows how to cook.

What did he do that was so special? He cut up potatoes, carrots, and parsnips, tossed them with a little extra-virgin olive oil and salt, and put them on a rimmed baking sheet in the oven next to a chicken he was roasting at 400°F. Honestly, I had never had vegetables that tasted so sweet! Roasting them at a high temperature caramelized the natural sugar in the vegetables. Do you notice something about the word "caramelized"? It has that lovely candy word "caramel" as its root. I was in LOVE with his vegetables (and, eventually, him too).

There are many recipes for roasted vegetables in this book, including broccoli, asparagus, cauliflower, Brussels sprouts, mushrooms, and acorn squash. They all make vegetables sing instead of fall flat.

You absolutely must try roasting some vegetables as soon as possible. Check out the recipes starting on page 191 for instructions and spice combinations for different vegetables. For example, I add a tiny bit of sugar to my broccoli to take away that bitter kick. Roasting vegetables will change your life.

My Stove Has Cobwebs Because I Don't Have Time to Make Breakfast, Lunch, or Dinner

Do you use your oven to store your tax documents or perhaps some canned goods? I first learned about this phenomenon when my oven stopped working two weeks before Thanksgiving and I had to call a repairman. I asked him about the upcoming holiday and he told me he *never* celebrates Thanksgiving because it is one of his busiest days. It seems that people turn on their ovens for the first time in a year on Thanksgiving morning, and then, uh-oh! It doesn't work! They call the repairman and he shows up and saves the day (and makes a big overtime bonus).

I am not going to say that there aren't times when takeout is necessary. One good friend tells this funny story of how her newly widowed mother tried to feed three kids and hold down a full-time job. One day she brought home a bucket of fried chicken, put it in the oven to warm up, and forgot about it until the smoke alarm went off. After grabbing the bucket out of the oven and putting out the flames in the sink, her kids ate the charred wet chicken (and teased their mother about it for years).

Most of us aren't having a crisis of this magnitude in our lives. We have just been conditioned to pick up the phone, stop at the drive-through, or run to Applebee's when we can't get it together to cook. Yes, we are time-strapped, but we also don't make cooking a priority. There is no shortcut here. If you want to be healthier, you need to put your tax documents in a filing cabinet and get that stove cleaned up and functioning.

Is this going to be easy? Heck no, especially if you are used to not cooking anything five to seven nights per week. This is a habit that will be challenging to break because it is easier to get takeout than to cook. You don't have to shop, chop, or do the dreaded scullery maid job of washing pots and pans.

However, there are instant benefits to cooking. First, there is weight loss, which will just happen because you are in control of how much cheese and how many sticks of butter you use in your food. Second, there is money in your bank account, which you can use for important things like vacations. It costs a family of four $28 on average to eat at McDonald's. Most of the meals in this book can be made for a lot less. Finally, there is the satisfaction of knowing that you fed yourself and perhaps your family or friends something healthy and delicious.

Some nights I am so tired I can hardly keep my head from hitting the kitchen table, but I look around and I am proud that I cooked something for my family. I know it is corny, but I expressed love when I made the meal and served it. There are many days when this meal is my biggest achievement.

Why Should I Cook? It Is Only Me

One of the main reasons people don't cook is that they don't want to waste time and money cooking a big meal for one (or two). Hopefully by now, I have convinced you that you need to cook for your health, but there are even better reasons.

A friend of mine who is a widow started putting out a cloth napkin, lighting a candle, and turning off her phone when she ate dinner. She realized that making a meal for herself was a gift, not a burden. Her meals would frequently serve four, and she got to be an expert at freezing the leftovers for nights when she was pressed for time.

Just because you are alone doesn't mean that you shouldn't take the time to enjoy your meal. Fill your home with lovely smells of cooking, turn off the screens, and enjoy the flavors, textures, and colors of the food you choose to cook. Food not only nourishes your body, it nourishes your soul. Take the time to cook for yourself; you deserve it.

Cooking Made Easier

As boring as grocery shopping and cooking healthy meals may be, this new skill requires some planning. I am sure you have heard this before, but you *must* think ahead. If you don't, you will end up dialing for takeout because you ran out of food. The good news is that I am sure you already have food in your pantry and refrigerator that can be turned into breakfast, lunches, and dinners. One of the features of Snack Girl recipes that my readers love is that they usually already have most, if not all, the ingredients in their homes, and every recipe in this book can be sourced from their local grocery store (pantry list, page 116). While I'm a fan of both Whole Foods and Trader Joe's, you don't *need* to shop there to get your healthy on.

Breakfast

I don't know about you, but my rear hasn't touched a chair at breakfast for a long time. I eat breakfast while I'm doing a bunch of other stuff for my family; with two kids I'm always running around, finding shoes, listening to complaints, fixing lunches, and wondering if we are going to make it out the door on time. My partner helps out quite a bit (that man can pack a backpack blindfolded with one hand tied behind his back), but I am still struggling to make the morning deadline.

> **EASY BREAKFASTS FOR HECTIC MORNINGS**
>
> Van's waffles
>
> Ezekiel or Alvarado Bakery sprouted bread with natural peanut butter
>
> Cheese sticks, handful of almonds, apple
>
> Fage yogurt
>
> KIND bar

What to do? My solution is to make some breakfast items ahead of time to be ready for the morning onslaught. Sometimes I cook several things on my day off, or I make breakfast the night before, while I am cooking dinner. If you really like the recipes, which you will, then you will find a way to create your own new cooking habits.

I include recipes for a couple of muffins, make-ahead pancake batter, and a very popular cereal bar (page 132). One of my favorites is just an egg, bread, and cheese combo that is baked in a muffin tin (page 138). Heat up one of those babies in the morning and you will not be stopping for that scone from Starbucks or the Egg Mc-Muffin at McDonald's.

Dinner

Dinner, for me at least, is the beast. At the end of my day I frequently want to lie facedown on the floor and not move. Instead of grinding my face into the carpet, I start heating pans and getting out my knife and cutting board. Do I find this relaxing? No. I still want to stop moving and get someone else to cook. I am lucky that I have a partner who is an exceptional cook and who hustles in the kitchen half the time. The other half, it is all me.

How do I do it? I have a plan. I put my blinders on and I execute. When things are truly crazy, I know that I have five meals I can pull out of my pantry on any given night; you'll find these and a shopping list on pages 119–120. These meals will beat takeout in a race to your table. On my fridge is a pad of paper so if I use up one of the key ingredients, I put it on the list and pick it up the next time I go to the store. I can't tell you how many times this plan has stopped me from calling the delivery guy.

Leftovers and frozen premade meals are a big part of my dinner strategy. Plenty of the meals in the recipe section can be made ahead, put in containers, and reheated when necessary. If cooking for yourself, making extra food and freezing it is a great way to save time. Plastic and glass containers come in almost limitless shapes and sizes so you can freeze single or family-size servings of your favorite meals. I have an extra freezer in my basement (because I have the space) so I can store meals to defrost for crazy nights.

My other secret weapon is my slow cooker; there is nothing more relaxing than walking in the door to a meal that is already cooked. Slow cookers come in a variety of styles and prices. Since I am feeding a family of four, I got the large oval (six-quart) size. It isn't fancy but it holds a constant temperature and is easy to clean. Get one with an insert you can remove for easy setup and cleaning. (If you're buying second-hand, double check! The older versions didn't have inserts.)

I think what stops many people from using their slow cooker is that you have to set it up in the morning to have dinner at night (remember how hard it is to get out the door in the morning—argh). I finally figured out that the night before I want to make something for my slow cooker, I can put all the ingredients in the ceramic insert, cover it, and leave it in the fridge. In the morning, I pop the insert into the cooker, cover it, turn it on, and walk away.

Why is this a brilliant idea?

1. **I cook on one night and I get two meals.** The slow cooker meal is prepared for the next night.

2. **Cleanup also happens only on one night.** When I use my slow cooker, I only have to wash the plates and the one pot. Hooray!

3. **My stress level the day of my slow cooker meal is much lower.** Because dinner is already made, I can take time to smell the roses when I get home.

No Cooking Required and Still Eating Well

After advocating for cooking for the last couple of pages, I am going to tell you a secret. When I don't have my family around to feed, I don't cook. This isn't to say that I don't eat healthy food or I start hitting the drive-through for breakfast. While I may not make a three-course meal for myself, I have become an expert at putting a few ingredients together quickly without turning on my oven or getting out my big kitchen knife to make a delicious snack (hence the name Snack Girl). Some of my readers have informed me that they put together a few of my snacks to make meals.

For example, I take a slice of 100 percent whole-grain bread, a little mustard, a slice of tomato, and an ounce of cheese and grill it under the broiler for a couple of minutes. Or I slice up an apple, spread on some peanut butter, and grab some whole-wheat crackers. Snack-Girl.com has a bunch of simple ideas like this to make it easy to stop grabbing a bag of chips or a cookie and start eating healthier. Check out the snacks section (page 219) and Snack-Girl.com for inspiration.

My Family Won't Get on the Healthy Train and Eat New Foods

How adventurous are you? I have a friend who won't touch a raw tomato and thinks seafood is disgusting, while I inhale raw oysters with glee. My six-year-old, on the other hand, thinks macaroni and cheese should be served at every meal. As a parent, I am constantly challenged to create meals that everyone in the family will eat. I have heard the same complaints from my readers: "My husband only likes meat and potatoes." Or "I am trying to get healthier but I end up cooking two (or more!) meals."

I hear you. This problem can really stop you from making the changes necessary to become healthier. The people who surround you exert an enormous influence on your choices. My dream for you is that you have a friend or relative who is solidly in your corner and helps you make the shift. I had that person in my husband, the vegetable roaster, and I am grateful for his support. What do you do if you don't have someone to help you?

You are just going to have to look in the mirror and support yourself. You don't have to lecture your sister about the 500-calorie muffins with 10 grams of saturated fat that she just devoured in seconds. Start nurturing yourself with good food and do your best to feel good about it.

Your children are the most impressionable when it comes to food choices. You can teach them all you want about healthy eating with your words, but your actions are what they will ultimately learn from. I've met mothers who have private candy stashes hidden from their kids. Why? Are they afraid that showing them their love of candy is going to ruin their children? Why not just teach them how to eat candy in moderation?

At a Weight Watchers meeting I talked with a father who joked about how his fresh blueberries keep disappearing because his son eats them. This is a great example of how his shift to healthier eating has had an impact on his family. He has a missing blueberry problem instead of a missing Doritos problem; that's a good problem to have. My advice is to choose to model healthy eating and then hope everyone follows.

On the other hand, you shouldn't make it hard for your family to follow you. Don't start serving lentil loaf or grilled tofu and declaring that everyone has to eat it.

If you want to turn people on to healthy eating, you are going to start with the meals that they love and tweak them a wee bit. My son eats my lighter macaroni and cheese with cauliflower (page 176) without noticing that I've changed the recipe. Is it the healthiest recipe ever? No, but it is much better than the boxed version of mac and cheese and he loves it. On taco night I serve a mixture of lean ground beef, corn, and mushrooms (page 154). Do I serve the glorified chips (aka taco shells)? Yep, but I eat one and then start putting my taco fixings on lettuce. My kids didn't even notice the difference in the filling.

Using meat as a flavoring agent instead of the center of the plate is a great trick for getting people to eat vegetables without putting up a big fight. When I started playing with this idea, I was amazed at how little meat you need to make something taste, well, *meaty*. Three things happen when you use less meat.

1. **Your meals cost less per serving** because meat costs more than beans and vegetables.

2. **You eat less saturated fat,** which is good for your heart.

3. **The calorie density (that is, the calories per serving) of your food decreases dramatically.**

Meat is not only expensive but also has a ton of calories when you compare it to, say, mushrooms. A pound of 80 percent lean ground beef has 1,152 calories, and a pound of mushrooms has 100 calories. A dramatic difference, isn't it? You get the same amount of filling for your taco but fewer calories, more fiber, and bonus micronutrients. This is such a simple way to shift everyone to healthier eating, and you don't even have to tell anyone you are doing it.

Don't make a big announcement about how you changed the taco filling or added veggies to the mac and cheese; just do it. If you set yourself up for confrontation, that is what you'll get. Ideally, mealtime should be peaceful; if your family doesn't eat the new healthy food that you cooked, just let it go. Whatever you do, do not get up and cook them something else (or you might never get them to eat anything new). It can take up to twelve times of introducing a new food for a child to even try it. Keep your expectations very low and keep modeling eating healthy. Eventually, they will come around.

I understand how emotional it can be to try to get someone you love to eat healthier. For example, I once worked for an hour making a special cheese sauce for my daughter's broccoli in an attempt to get her to eat some. She didn't even touch it! I felt like a failure when I was actually a success because my heart was in the right place.

Don't give up. Just keep trying new things and good stuff will happen.

Everyday Temptations

Coworkers Keep Bringing in Cookies and I Can Smell Them from My Desk

Are you aware of how much free food you are offered on a daily basis? It is a bit scary once you calculate how much comes your way. The office environment used to get me into a lot of trouble. There was a candy bowl on my route to and from the copier. How many times a day would I pass it? Probably about ten, and every time I walked by, I would think about having a piece.

One of the first things I noticed when I walked into my editor's office was the candy bowl she had perched on a shelf. Here I am, attempting to represent a book on healthy eating, and all I can think about is the candy bowl! I spent part of the meeting actively avoiding the Dove chocolate she probably didn't remember was there.

Then there were the bagels and pastries that appeared at morning business meetings. I would eat breakfast, go to work, and be faced with yet another breakfast. What was this company trying to do to me? I would sit there staring at a cheese danish for an hour as people droned on. Do you think I managed to convince myself that I didn't want it? Or did I rationalize my consumption by telling myself I would eat less lunch or do an extra mile on the treadmill?

Treadmill.

Now that I work for myself, I have fewer temptations—except when I volunteer in my community. At my children's school, there is a monthly coffee with the principal, bake sales, and parent organization meetings, all with coffee cake, brownies, boxes of pizza, cookies, and doughnuts. I serve on a nonprofit board where inevitably I am sitting in front of a plate of freshly baked banana bread.

The issue isn't that people share goodies. The issue is the *number* of them that I am offered. I think the people who bring in their favorite baked goods to share are trying to do something nice for their coworkers. The receptionist with the candy bowl was trying to make us smile as we did battle with the aging copy machine. The problem is that most of this stuff (how come no one puts out a plate of carrots, celery sticks, and hummus at a meeting?) is simply a lot of empty calories. How are they empty? They are devoid of many nutrients we need to function. For example, if you eat a medium carrot, you munch down 35 calories and 270 percent of your daily value of vitamin A. If you eat a brownie, 330 calories later you supplied your body with 25 percent of your daily vitamin A. Vitamin A is just one of the nutrients that a carrot provides, but you can see right away the calorie cost for all that nutrition is much lower with the carrot than the brownie. Most of us can't eat a lot of calorie-dense and nutrient-light food (aka junk food) and maintain a reasonable waistline. Unfortunately, most of us can't turn down the crap either.

Reality Bites

I once visited a meditation center where you could wear a feather around your neck to signal that you were on a silent retreat. The people around you took care of you by leaving you entirely alone. Wouldn't it be cool if you could wear a cookie sign with a slash through it and no one would offer you any sweets? The sign would let people know, "It's not about you. It's about me!! You are helping me by *not* offering a treat." On days when you felt like having a cookie, you could not wear the sign. Life would be so easy if we lived in meditation retreat centers.

What about willpower? Can't you "just say no" to all that food?

Every time I walk by that candy jar, a little part of my brain says, "You need some of that." My body craves the salty and sugary hit of the mini Snickers bar, and while I am able to walk by once and deny my impulse, after ten times, I am powerless and I can no longer resist.

Forget physical cravings for a minute—how about the fact that it is considered rude to turn down a food gift. I mean, how ungrateful are you? This person is trying so hard to do something nice for you and you just said, "No, thank you." I always feel bad when someone offers me something nice and I don't take it. The people who will really get to you are the ones in your family. These relatives love you and want to show their love by feeding you, whether you are hungry or not. If you don't accept their offer of food, guess what? You just turned down their token of love and they might feel rejected or even angry with you. Sheesh.

But the road to healthy eating isn't comfortable. You've got to find an answer to all this free food that will support your goals without hurting anyone's feelings. Your relationship to others is important, but so is nourishing yourself. **You have to start to get comfortable with the uncomfortable.** No, it isn't comfortable to sit staring at a cheese danish for an hour in a meeting, or telling your mother "No, thank you" for the tenth time when she offers you her homemade cake, but it takes some strength to lose weight and feel good.

How to Cope with the Avalanche of Free Food

Your first step is to get a handle on your treat consumption by writing it down. In "Healthy Weight and Healthy Image," I talked about food journaling (page 20), a powerful tool for recording and understanding your entire food intake. Unfortunately, most of us find food journaling to be tedious. I suggest you start by writing down only your *treats* on a daily basis. Get a small notepad and put it in your purse, briefcase, or backpack or just use a notepad app on your phone. Every time you eat a treat, write it down. What is a treat? Here are a few examples:

NOT TREAT	TREAT
Coffee	Mocha Frappuccino
Regular hamburger	½ pound hamburger with cheese, bacon, mayo
Oatmeal	Homemade oatmeal cookies
Carrot sticks	Bag of potato chips
Scrambled eggs	Doughnut

I know there are people who are convinced that their homemade air-popped popcorn with a little Mrs. Dash is a treat. For most people, the popcorn is a drop in the bucket compared to the bag of Doritos they just inhaled. Obviously, you have to define your treats, but I am making the assumption that you know when you are in "calorie bomb" territory.

Why write it down every time you indulge? An amazing thing happens when you start to make yourself accountable. First, you might turn down the stale bag of Chips Ahoy in your car if you think about having to type "stale Chips Ahoy" on your phone. Second, you get a record of what you have eaten for the day. For example, while my children are screaming *"Dessert!"* at the top of their lungs, I will check out my notepad to remember if I had that chocolate peanut butter cookie with my coffee today or yesterday before I join them. My memory isn't that great and I tend to selectively forget my indulgences until it is too late. My goal is to try to eat just one treat per day, so I will forgo dessert if I had something sweet earlier and try to remember the experience so I don't feel deprived.

Now that you have assessed your treat consumption, what is your goal? That is entirely up to you. If you are at five treats per day, you could start by limiting yourself to four. I don't think a wholesale denial of goodies is going to help you stop eating them on a long-term basis.

Do not go cold turkey! I tried this once and found myself on a Ben & Jerry's bender a few days later. Love yourself, acknowledge your love of junk food, and allow yourself to eat it—just eat less of it.

What is going to happen? You will start to get straTREATic (like strategic—yes, I made up my own word). You will find that you no longer want to eat the crappy Chips Ahoy because you are saving up for something really good, like homemade chocolate chip cookies. Certain pleasures are too special to turn down, so enjoy them. You can feel self-righteous when you manage to avoid the candy that you sort of like and have that Mocha Frappuccino that you really crave with a friend. Now you are not mindlessly eating all the junk food that comes your way—you are making choices! Don't tell anyone you are doing this, and if someone says you are being "good," tell them that you are saving up for that pint of beer or whatever indulgence you have in mind. Another good strategy when dealing with people who want to give you a food gift is to be honest: "I'm not going to have that brownie you offered me now, because later I am going to my mother's birthday party and my dad made his special chocolate cake." No one is going to be angry with you for being straTREATic. Instead, they will admire your planning and maybe even be compassionate enough to support you in your choice.

My personal goal is one treat per day, and I can usually stick to it as long as it isn't the holidays. While I don't look like a supermodel (and never have), I maintain a healthy weight without feeling deprived. I am convinced that if I stopped all treat consumption, I would be thinner. But for me, being thinner isn't as important as enjoying my life, and that includes my sweet, salty, and bubbly pleasures.

Treats and Children

When you have kids, you start to view treats with new eyes. Some of us start off not wanting our children to have any candy or added sugar. Others want to give their children everything because they were deprived as children. For partners who share parenting responsibilities, there can be big disagreements about the amount of candy, junk food, soda, and cookies their children eat.

I have received e-mails from my readers about what to bring for "soccer snacks" because other parents bring sugary packaged snacks and juice boxes. What happened to bananas or quartered oranges and water? Just as you may work for a company that keeps a kitchen stocked with tempting snacks, your children are constantly around a pile of tasty low-quality food. Should you forbid your child from eating any of it? I heard of a San Francisco mother who decided her daughter wasn't going to have birthday cake at parties because of the sugar. That lasted until the kid was about three years old. You can't teach your children moderation if the message is "Just say no to all sugary treats."

My parents never brought candy or sugary cereals into the house. I would marvel at the Twinkies in other kids' lunch boxes and wish I could have them. When I was eleven I had a job as a mother's helper for the grand salary of $2 per hour. The minute I got paid I spent that money on Snickers bars and a Coca-Cola habit that my parents didn't even know about.

In my current household, where my husband and I have some control over what our children ingest, I have tried to remain reasonable. Many days before dinner has been served my children have managed to get their hands on a treat. In Ellyn Satter's parenting book *How to Get Your Kid to Eat: But Not Too Much*, she stresses that parents are responsible for what food is presented to their children and the manner in which it is presented. Children are responsible for how much or even whether they eat. I took her advice and I do my best to present healthy meals and hope my kids eat them. I don't use dessert as a reward because most of the time during the day they have already eaten a dessert at school. If I ask, "Hey, did you have a birthday party at school today?" and they did, they don't get dessert after dinner.

What I am attempting to do is help them become aware of the amount of sweets they eat. Do I buy them candy? Yes. Do I make them cookies? Yes. But do we eat sugary cereal for breakfast, cupcakes at lunch, and ice cream after dinner? No. Do they bug me for more junk food? Absolutely, but I am consistent in my one-treat rule. They accept it 90 percent of the time, even if they test it all the time.

It Seems Like Every Day I'm Invited to Another Celebration

When I started writing Snack Girl, it seemed I was constantly giving my readers advice about avoiding food "land mines" at occasions like Super Bowl parties (could I suggest healthier snacks?), Fourth of July barbecues (are there any healthy hot dogs?), and Thanksgiving (how about some lighter side dishes?).

Then there are the everyday birthday parties, baby showers, and retirement dinners that we all find ourselves attending. If you count the holidays, it would be easy to be invited to one party per week. And if you have a large extended family, that number might be two per week. Having two chances per week to eat heavy food and drink a lot of alcohol is a big problem for those of us trying to be healthier. I've never been to a party where they served carrot juice and tofu. If the party is casual, then we have the ubiquitous chips, pizza, sheet cake, and beer. It's a calorie-bomb bonanza!

It's an impossible situation, too. Here you are surrounded by people who want you to enjoy yourself: "Hey, let me get you a drink. So glad you could make it. Try my latest version of onion dip." Yes, I want the drink and the onion dip and I want to be involved in the social interaction that is a party. I could never say, "Oh, onion dip, that has sour cream and onion soup mix, right? No, that isn't on my latest healthy eating plan. Can I just have a spring water, preferably from a green bottle?" My style is to grab the real drink and start tasting the onion dip with potato chips (not the carrot sticks).

How Do I Deal with All That Food?

First, let's deal with the food. How do we overindulge at parties? The free food and drinks are seemingly limitless and we often lose control for a number of reasons. We are having so much fun socializing we forget how many plates of salty, fatty, crunchy food we have chowed down. Or maybe there is someone or a situation that is making us feel uncomfortable and we start eating to overcome the stress of the event. How can you get this party under control?

First, do some research about the hoedown. Before you attend an event, ask the host or hostess what they are serving, then make a plan of what you will eat. All party hosts love to talk about their parties and they will be excited that you want to know about the food. If the party has cheese puffs, beef stew, red wine, and chocolate cake, decide right now that you will have three cheese puffs, one bowl of beef stew, a glass of red wine, and half a slice of chocolate cake. When that baked Brie shows up, well, that is just not on your plan. If you are lucky and raw or steamed vegetables (aka crudités) are part of the menu, fill your plate with half vegetables, just like you would at home.

Whatever you do, keep count of how many plates you have picked up and ask yourself before you pick up another one, if you are really hungry or just eating because the deep-fried calamari are your favorite.

I try to limit myself to whatever will fit on one small plate because you know that after you finish your one plate, people keep sharing their food with you. "Here, try one of these pumpkin muffins. I picked up two." Maybe I am too nice, but I can't turn someone down who hands me a muffin, or anything else they want to share for that matter. I always seem to eat more than I plan to at one of these events, and I suspect you do too.

If dessert is being served, and you are anything like me, you are having some dessert. I always ask for half a slice of whatever is being served. I say something like, "Wow, that looks so good! Can I have just half a slice? I pigged out on the onion dip. What a great party."

Finally, if you have a choice about what you are served, choose carefully. I have been stuck at a rubber-chicken wedding, looking longingly at the vegetarian entrée that a friend of mine asked for ahead of time. When you cruise the buffet, check out the whole table (or tables), then go back to the beginning of the line and pick out the food you like the best. I went to this top-notch party in San Francisco and all I had was champagne, sushi, and some great moves on the dance floor. I felt like a million bucks, didn't overindulge, and had a wonderful time.

What to Drink? The Liquid Calorie Problem

What is the first thing that happens when you walk into a party? Either you declare, "I need a drink!" or someone hands you one as soon as you take off your coat. The average American consumes between 140 and 180 calories of sugary drinks per day without even attending a party. These are calories we enjoy, but they lack any nutrition and contribute to our widening waistlines.

Parties are difficult. You have to handle not only the temptation of the variety of drinks, but also the social pressure. Have you ever tried to say "No thanks, I'm not thirsty" at a party? *Everyone* has a drink in his or her hand. Recently, I confronted this problem at my twenty-fifth high school reunion. My best friend and I had gone out to dinner and shared a bottle of wine, so by the time I reached the reunion I was feeling giggly. After we arrived, the first thing I did was order a drink to fit in with the rest of my class. After that drink, I realized that I couldn't feel my feet. What to do? I asked the bartender for a glass of water with ice in a nice-looking glass. What tickled me was that people kept asking me what I was drinking. "Hey, that looks good. What is it?" Ummm, water? They thought I had a vodka tonic or something fun when I was just rehydrating so I wouldn't fall down. What I realized from this experience is that the perception of "having a drink" is much more important than the reality.

Now that we agree that you must have a drink in your hand, what are your choices? If you like drinking soda, try to limit yourself to one, then switch to water. I like getting a bubbly mineral water or seltzer with lime because it satisfies my need for bubbles with zero calories. If you hate seltzer alone, try diluting juice with the seltzer. This is particularly refreshing with orange or cranberry juice with a slice of lime, and (bonus!) it looks like a real drink.

If you are trying to lose weight and you drink alcohol, you will have to confront the fact that alcohol has a lot of empty calories. When I began reading diet books, I always flipped to the section on alcohol to learn how much I could drink and still lose weight.

Here is a strategy from Cynthia Sass's *Cinch! Conquer Cravings, Drop Pounds, and Lose Inches*:

I haven't included an "alcohol allowance" on this plan because alcohol isn't essential for health, and research shows that even moderate drinking—one drink a day—can increase the risk of breast cancer.

Man, what a buzz kill! She advises that if you must have a drink, allow yourself one drink per day—but only after completing thirty days on her plan.

Joel Fuhrman, who wrote the bestselling *Eat to Live*, says in his alcohol section:

Moderate drinking has been associated with a lower incidence of coronary heart disease in more than forty prospective studies.

Hooray! But, he then goes on to explain how alcohol is also associated with increased fat around the waist. Uh-oh. His conclusion:

It is much wiser to avoid the detrimental effects of alcohol completely and protect yourself from heart disease with nutritional excellence.

He, too, advises one drink a day, but only if it will help you stay on his healthy plan.

Here we are at a party, and leading diet and health experts are telling us to have one drink. If you are starting to unwind and, perhaps, shaking your booty, one drink isn't going to cut it.

When you start to tune in to how many calories are in different alcoholic drinks, you can make informed choices regarding how you want to indulge. For example, sugary piña coladas and slushy margaritas are not the same as a 4-ounce glass of wine in terms of calories. The sweet mixed drinks are calorie bombs and should be consumed as treats, like dessert. There are potentially 740 calories in a 10-ounce frozen margarita. Yikes!

The good news is that champagne (or sparkling wine) has about 90 calories per 4-ounce glass, so if you are at a super swanky party and they are handing this out, don't feel bad about drinking it. If I am going to a casual party and it is acceptable to bring drinks, I pick up a six-pack of my favorite light beer (Corona Light) for myself and something nicer for the host.

How many drinks should you have? That's up to you. What I do know is that you

AVERAGE CALORIES IN COMMON ALCOHOLIC DRINKS

1 glass (5 ounces) red wine	106 calories
1 glass (5 ounces) white wine	100 calories
1 bottle (12 ounces) beer (such as Budweiser)	146 calories
Rum and Coke (7 ounces)	180 calories
Gin and tonic (7 ounces)	189 calories
Jack Daniel's on the rocks (1.5 ounces whisky)	98 calories

have to watch how much you consume if you want to lose weight. My strategy is less a daily strategy than a weekly strategy. I try to limit the days that I drink to Friday, Saturday, and Sunday and have no more than two drinks a day. If I know that I am going to a party on Wednesday, then I drop a weekend drinking day. I have lost weight when I manage to employ this strategy consistently. The holidays make it much harder to stay on plan, but I keep trying.

My other strategy is never to order a sugary, slushy drink at a bar or party. I'd rather fire up my own blender or get out my martini shaker. The three recipes that follow, which use fresh lime or lemon juice and agave syrup, are tasty, lower-calorie alternatives for those in love with the sweeter drinks.

If you don't have a glass or plastic juicer, buy one. It takes about thirty seconds to slice a lime in half and juice it.

The agave syrup can be found next to the honey in your grocery store. It is pricey, but it makes great-tasting drinks. You will never go back to premade mix after you try it mixed with fresh juice.

Finally, I like to use a metal cocktail shaker to mix my drink. You get some exercise shaking it and the taste is much improved by shaking it with ice and then pouring it through a strainer. (You look cool, too.) I have found cocktail shakers at my local Target. Please feel free to use a spoon to mix your drink if you don't have a shaker.

Relax Your Mind Margarita

You can relax your mind because you just saved yourself a bunch of calories.

Serves 1

½ lime

1 ½ ounces tequila

2 teaspoons agave syrup

Ice cubes

1 lime wedge (optional)

Kosher salt (optional)

Juice the lime half in a hand juicer and pour into a cocktail shaker or glass. Add the tequila, agave syrup, and ice cubes and mix well.

Strain carefully into a glass and enjoy.

Optional: If you like salt on the rim of your glass, first run a wedge of lime along the rim. Pour salt into a small dish and rub the rim of the glass in the salt. Be sure to pour the margarita into the center of the glass.

158 calories | 0 g fat | 0 g saturated fat | 13.9 g carbohydrates
10.8 g sugar | 0.2 g protein | 0 g fiber | 0 mg sodium

Lemon Drop Martini

1 slice of lemon

Granulated sugar

Ice cubes

1 ounce vodka

½ ounce Triple Sec or other orange liqueur

1 tablespoon plus 1 teaspoon freshly squeezed lemon juice

1 teaspoon agave syrup

This drink should be served with some sugar on the rim of the martini glass. Run a lemon slice around the rim of the glass so the sugar will stick. Pour some sugar on a small plate and rub the rim of the glass in the sugar.

Fill a cocktail shaker or another glass half full with ice. Add the vodka, Triple Sec, lemon juice, and agave syrup and mix until extremely cold. Carefully pour through a strainer into the center of the martini glass and enjoy!

140 calories | 0 g fat | 0 g saturated fat | 11.7 g carbohydrates
11.7 g sugar | 0 g protein | 0 g fiber | 0 mg sodium

Pineapple Vodka Slushie

Put the ice cubes in the blender and pulse until crushed. Add the pineapple, vodka, Triple Sec, and agave syrup (if using) and blend until frothy. Pour into a margarita glass and enjoy.

Serves 1

3 ice cubes

¼ cup crushed pineapple in 100% unsweetened pineapple juice

1 ounce vodka

½ ounce Triple Sec or other orange liqueur

½ teaspoon agave syrup (optional)

154 calories | 0 g fat | 0 g saturated fat | 11.3 g carbohydrates
18.4 g sugar | 0.5 g protein | 0.5 g fiber | 50 mg sodium

Going Out to Restaurants Without Wearing an Elastic Waistband

Have you noticed how your pants feel much tighter if you go out to one of our nation's restaurants? I'm talking about the Chili's, Applebee's, and Olive Gardens in every large and midsized town in America. Under the 2010 health care law (aka Obamacare), these chains are required to list calorie information on their menus. The calorie numbers have shocked me over and over again when I go to one of these places. Shiner Bock Ribs at Chili's boast 2,310 calories, Aussie Cheese Fries at Outback Steakhouse have 2,134 calories, and a Bella Burger at Ruby Tuesday's rings up 1,145 calories. Needless to say, if you are a frequent visitor to these places you need a strategy.

The wonderful thing about having the calorie amount at your fingertips is that you can make lighter choices. All of the big chains now have menu items that feature less fat and fewer calories. Applebee's even lists Weight Watchers PointsPlus on its menu. I have ordered a 4-ounce steak at Outback, skipped the fries, and had a salad and been perfectly content. You can add a plain or sweet baked potato if you like.

But what if you *want* the ribs?

Instruct your waiter to pack up half of your order before he even brings it to the table. I learned this strategy from a sandwich maker at Subway who informed me, "That food would kill me if I didn't take half of it home." This brilliant guy was employing this strategy before the health care law went into effect and getting two meals for one!

Most restaurants are not required to list nutritional information on their menus and you cannot interrogate the manager under a hot light about the calorie content of the food. What you can do is ask for your food to be cooked and served in a way that supports your healthy goals. Here are some perfectly reasonable requests that a restaurant (including a chain) will fulfill for you:

- Put the dressing on the side
- No bread or chip basket for the table
- Grill rather than deep-fry the entrée
- Substitute a side salad for the fries

These four simple requests will save you hundreds of calories every time you go out to eat and you will find that waitstaff are happy to make changes for you. I learned this the hard way after a post on Snack-Girl.com criticized a local restaurant for the lack of fresh food in the kid's meal. After the post appeared, the manager called me up and told me that I could have had fresh fruit instead of fries if I had just asked for it.

Who knew?

I shared this information with my readers and many of them were surprised by how far a restaurant will go to make you something other than what is on the menu. Of course, some readers were already hip to ordering substitutions and changes, and were wondering what cave I live in.

The lesson here is that you can ask for all sorts of changes to the menu and you will get what you want. You are not causing a scene or drawing attention to yourself by being picky. My husband always asks for water with no ice, which I think is ridiculous, and the waitstaff always gets it for him. If he can do that, you can ask for the shrimp to be grilled and not deep-fried.

My Car Drives Itself to the Drive-Through

Close your eyes for a second and imagine your drive to work, school, or wherever you go on a daily basis. Maybe you are lucky and get to walk or ride your bike to your destination.

Think about all the places that you pass and ask yourself how many of them beckon to you. I live in a rural neighborhood and it takes me all of six minutes to drive to my office, during which I pass a Dunkin' Donuts drive-through and a Cumberland Farms convenience store.

Every time I pass these stores, I think about going in and getting a doughnut or a sweet coffee drink. It is like the candy bowl on the receptionist's desk. Usually, I am passing them when I am feeling a little hungry and there, in neon, is my solution. These places smell good and they offer something quick and delicious all for under $2. How can I resist? We all have the drinks and snacks that we love at these places no matter how much we want to avoid processed foods.

For example, I have a friend who is a triathlete who goes on and on about the

Shamrock Shake at McDonald's, which she passes on her way to and from work. My brilliant friend Bridget cannot get her morning coffee at Starbucks without her maple oat pecan scone. My downfall is doughnuts, and I know where all the best ones are within a ten-mile radius. How I love you, jelly doughnut from the little bakery on my drive into town . . .

Let's call these stops that we make "Junk Food Drive-Buys," or JFDB. If you want to lose weight, you have got to get a handle on your JFDB. The problem is that even before you go by the junk food treat that you love, you have already decided to have it.

My first wake-up call to these habits was analyzing how many calories were in my favorite JFDB. What I found was scary.

When I first took a look at my JFDB, I realized that I was kidding myself about the impact of these "little" snacks on my health; I was adding hundreds of calories to my day and not even considering how much they would impact my waistline. Part of the reason was that few of the foods I was picking up had nutrition labels (like a cookie from a local café). Without that information, it was easier to rationalize my JFDB.

Once I confronted reality (ouch!), I knew I had to stop habitually eating this stuff, but I loved it. I had to ask myself one hard question: "Can I drive by the drive-buy?"

I know this sounds obvious, but for some of us (like me), this is hard. I know how I felt, which was pissed off that I couldn't have my treat. I *need* my JFDB!!!

My solution was to have a super yummy, alternative healthier snack in my purse or backpack that I liked more than the JFDB. When I have a small bag of cinnamon sugar almonds (page 270), I don't have to stop and spend $2 on a cookie. Snack-Girl.com has a bunch of simple,

CALORIES AND GRAMS OF FAT IN JUNK FOOD DRIVE-BUYS

Glazed doughnut	200 calories 12 grams of fat
2-ounce bag of Doritos	280 calories 16 grams of fat
McD's Peppermint Mocha (12 ounces)	340 calories 12 grams of fat
Starbucks maple oat pecan scone	440 calories 18 grams of fat
Subway chocolate chip cookie	210 calories 10 grams of fat
McD's Shamrock Shake (12 ounces)	530 calories 15 grams of fat

easy, affordable ideas for snacks that are healthy, have only 100 to 150 calories, and taste better than the JFDB. I've included ten sweet and ten savory snacks on pages 223–226.

The JFDB that include high-calorie coffee drinks can be replaced with lower-calorie coffee drinks if you know how to order. Ordering a small, using nonfat milk, and skipping the whipped cream are steps that will minimize the calorie impact. Starbucks has some sugar-free syrups made with stevia that aren't bad. I stopped ordering sugar-filled lattes when I realized that what I really love is coffee. A cup of coffee has only 2 calories, and when I add 2 tablespoons of whole milk with a teaspoon of sugar, the entire drink has less than 60 calories.

Take Care of Yourself

If you are in the mind-set that you deserve your JFDB and they make your day go easier, you have to realize that you are taking care of a need for sugar, fat, and comfort, but you aren't nourishing your body.

Planning ahead with something truly healthy and delicious is a way to be kind to yourself. I know Oprah and others advocate bubble baths and soft pajamas, but the work of buying and preparing some food is key to a healthier and happier you. It isn't a chore to cook and pack little containers of delicious, healthy snacks if you tune in to the gift you are giving yourself.

Breaking a JFDB habit is hard, but as you slowly let go of it, you will feel better. You'll discover that apples and peanut butter or homemade kettle corn (page 242) can satisfy your need for crunch and sweetness. Maybe you will never give up your favorite junk food, and that is okay, but you will find that it doesn't taste as good after you start eating food that actually nourishes your body.

A freshly made doughnut will taste great every once in a while if you don't mindlessly eat one *every day*. My suggestion is to buy that doughnut, take two slow bites, and savor it. Some people will be amazed that they needed only two bites to be satisfied and can toss the rest of the confection to the birds. Others love it so much that they eat the whole thing. Whatever you do, don't beat yourself up for loving a doughnut once in a while. Just be active in your choice to eat it.

Emotional Eating

The subject of eating in response to emotions rather than hunger is a difficult one to tackle. Whenever I approach this subject on Snack Girl, I always get a couple of e-mails that tell me I have no idea what I am talking about. The responses are along these lines:

> Your post makes it seem as if this problem can just go away by tuning in to my feelings. I've tried everything and I can't stop eating. Don't try to tell me how easy it is to stop my out-of-control behavior. I can't do it!

My heart breaks for these people because I never mean to belittle their problems, and I always e-mail them back to tell them I wish I could help. There is a whole range of disordered eating and eating disorders that I cannot begin to address because I don't have the expertise. In this book, I will attempt to address "garden variety" emotional eating, which I define as a response to an immediate situation. My favorite resource on more problematic emotional eating is Geneen Roth. Her book *Breaking Free from Emotional Eating* is a great place to start. If you have deeper emotional food issues, I hope you will seek professional help.

Many of us are unconsciously eating too much as a way to deal with what we are feeling. I have met very few people who eat only when they are hungry. For example, my ultrasvelte husband never eats to feel better, but he will overindulge when he is celebrating. I tend to lose control when I am upset and need to be comforted. For example, after a recent argument with that same skinny husband, I drove directly to Friendly's and ordered the Jim Dandy sundae (the one with bananas, chocolate sauce, whipped cream, and three scoops of ice cream). I can also be found with a big bowl of potato chips at the end of the day if I have had a challenging day at work. If you are trying to get healthy, addressing why you eat when you're not hungry may go a long way toward helping you lose weight.

After a Stressful Day My Best Friends Are Ben & Jerry

Imagine this: You are driving your minivan on the highway when your two-year-old decides to unbuckle her seat belt. Just then, a large truck cuts you off and you hit the brakes as your child bounces onto the floor.

What do you do?

If you are my pal, Bonnie, you start driving ten miles below the speed limit, get off at the next exit, park the car and strap your child in her seat, wait ten seconds at every stop sign, and kiss the ground when you get out of the car. As you walk in your door, you cross yourself and then grab a spoon and a can of chocolate frosting. Bonnie's daughter was fine, a bit teary-eyed because her mother yelled at her, but Bonnie was shaking and the frosting calmed her down.

There is a very real correlation between stress and eating. After the incident on the highway, if we had sampled Bonnie's saliva, in addition to the frosting, we would have found a large amount of cortisol, a hormone released by the brain. Cortisol is our "fight or flight" hormone and its release is a natural, normal reaction to stress. Cortisol gives our brain a quick burst of energy by diverting available glucose to it to help it function. Many types of stressful situations in which we perceive a threat, such as an argument with a friend, a looming deadline, or an overwhelming to-do list, trigger cortisol release. Bonnie's cortisol infusion helped her react quickly and effectively to the truck cutting her off.

But there is a downside to cortisol.

When scientists inject cortisol into human subjects (sounds like fun, doesn't it?), they have demonstrated that cortisol is associated with increased appetite, cravings for sugar, and weight gain. And, get this, the sugary, fatty foods that we crave relieve the stress. Hello!

Our bodies rev up because we have encountered a freaked-out moment, and then our brain tells us to eat some sugar and fat because we burned a lot of energy when we dealt with the stressor.

In *The End of Overeating*, David Kessler outlines the body's response to salty, fatty, and sweet food (what he calls "highly palatable food"):

The neurons in the brain that are stimulated by taste and other properties of highly palatable food are part of the opioid circuitry, which is the body's primary pleasure system. The "opioids," also known as endorphins, are chemicals produced in the brain that have rewarding effects similar to drugs such as morphine and heroin . . . . The opioids produced by eating high-sugar, high-fat foods can relieve pain or stress and calm us down.

Or put more simply: Our bodies and brains react to that canned frosting or pint of ice cream the way they would to heroin. And what do we know about heroin? It is addictive.

Imagine all of us, cruising along, wanting to eat healthier, and slamming into stressful events that are out of our control. We toss all of our resolutions and plans out the window and succumb to our craving, and then what do we do? We feel guilty.

"Ohhh, how could I have taken out that frozen cheesecake? I ate half of it and I was saving it for my aunt's birthday. Why did my boss have to yell at me?"

You're concerned about keeping your job and you're mad at yourself for eating cheesecake. Everyone, even super healthy people, eats for reasons other than hunger some of the time. It's human! Look, life happens, bad things happen, and you have to give yourself a break. The chemicals in your brain are telling you to eat comfort food and it is impossible to change hardwired responses that have evolved over millions of years. None of us is strong enough to turn that system off.

So what are you going to do? You are going to have to evaluate the patterns of situations and emotions that cause you to overeat and determine what you can change. Keep in mind that this change isn't going to be instant. Changing habits that have been reinforced for years takes time and practice. But if your kid gets into a bicycle accident and you eat a mega chocolate chip cookie, forgive yourself and move on.

Replace the Comfort Food with Comfort Food

After not getting into a major accident on the freeway, my friend Bonnie could have grabbed some carrot sticks to calm her nerves instead of canned frosting. But who does that? Superwoman? Popeye? I don't know anyone who reaches for carrots when they are upset. Somehow raw vegetables aren't comforting.

Why are comfort foods so comforting? There are a couple of reasons. Often comfort foods make you feel better because they remind you of a person or time in your life that was safe. For example, if a beloved grandmother made you chicken soup when you were sick, you might want that soup when you are feeling tense. Comfort foods usually have the carbohydrates (think pasta or potatoes) that the body craves as a response to the cortisol release. Finally, comfort foods go down easy. I'm not saying crunching on a carrot is stressful, but it definitely doesn't feel as nice as slurping down some hot, creamy macaroni and cheese.

When I argue with my husband my reaction is that I want a sundae. Yes, I will feel better if I have one, but what else could I eat? I decided that my new comfort food could be a BLT. The sandwich is a healthier choice than the sundae (even with a couple of slices of bacon). I find that it isn't as easy to eat as a sundae (more crunchy, less gooey), so I eat less of it if I'm not really that hungry. Having a BLT makes me feel calmer and I am able to speak without fumes coming out of my ears.

Take a good hard look at your go-to comfort foods. Are they ice cream, cookies, cake, candy, macaroni and cheese, or French fries? What if you could find comfort foods that are healthier for you? Since we are hardwired to eat when stressed, you will have more success if you eat for comfort when necessary, but change the foods that you turn to.

Here is a list of my favorite savory comfort foods:

1. Chicken noodle soup
2. Mashed Potatoes with Cauliflower (page 207)

3. Airy and Easy Mac and Cheese (page 176)

4. Slice of pizza with lots of vegetables

5. Homemade Skinny Fries (page 208)

6. Roasted Vegetable Quesadilla (page 205)

7. Chicken and Vegetable Potpie (page 184)

8. Mighty Meatloaf (page 186)

9. Sneaky Zucchini Lasagna (page 182)

10. Slow Cooker Beef Stew (page 161)

All of these comfort foods feature vegetables and all of them will give you both the calming effect your mind seeks and the nutrients your body needs.

For those of you who don't find savory foods comforting, the sweet category is a bit more difficult to make healthy. The first thing to do is to try to minimize the damage. As a teenager, I ate an entire pint of Ben & Jerry's Coffee Heath Bar Crunch after breaking it off with the latest boyfriend. Notice how I did the breaking up and still needed the ice cream. Could I have eaten less and still gotten comfort? Of course! But I had a spoon, the pint, and no one to share it with. What I needed was to put the ice cream in a small bowl. Also, I could have used a friend (with another small bowl) to share both my pint and my heartache of having hurt a lovely guy because I wanted to play with (yet another) boy toy. Teenagers!

Now when I want ice cream, I eat slow-churned chocolate with chocolate sauce in a bowl while sitting down. Slow-churned ice cream has two-thirds the calories and half the fat of regular ice cream with the same creamy, satisfying texture. For example, half a cup of Edy's Slow-Churned Chocolate has only 100 calories; compare that to Ben & Jerry's Chocolate Therapy at 240 calories. Sorry Ben & Jerry, you are officially fired as my shrink.

Try these ideas for taming your sweet comfort food habit:

1. ½ cup slow-churned ice cream

2. No-bake cookies (pages 251–256)

3. Hot, Thick, and Dark Chocolate Drink (page 272)

4. Square of dark chocolate

5. Fruit Popsicles or sorbet

6. Green Smoothie (page 232)
7. Greek yogurt with jam
8. Healthier Apple Crisp (page 267)
9. Instant Banana Pudding (page 268)
10. French toast, light on the maple syrup

Recognize your need for comfort food, embrace it, and make choices about what you are going to eat when you're stressed out. Buy and/or prepare your new comfort foods and have them ready to replace your old favorites. Allow yourself that comfort, because you deserve it. Just try to make a healthier version so that you nourish your body as well as soothe it.

I Need a Drink

Tired? Frustrated? Had the day from hell? How about a nice glass of wine? All that stress will just melt away in a puddle of tipsiness. As we all know, alcohol in the right amounts lowers blood pressure and heart rate and calms us down. Wouldn't it be great if it didn't have any other consequences? In "Everyday Temptations" I talk about how some healthy eating coaches believe that alcohol should be avoided (page 53). On the other hand, there is research showing that the phytochemicals in a glass of red or white wine can be good for you. If alcohol is your relaxation method of choice, you will benefit from knowing the number of calories you are drinking. Check out the list of drinks and calorie amounts on page 54.

When I was on Weight Watchers, I could stay within my point range for the day until it was time for my evening beer. It became crystal clear that my nightly brewski (or two) was holding me back from losing weight.

I had my ritual: Opening the beer, pouring it into the glass, and taking that first sip can be so lovely. I didn't want to give it up just to be thinner and healthier. Doesn't being healthy also mean being relaxed?

Since I didn't want to stop drinking beer, I made some changes. I started drinking light beer, cut my consumption to a few days a week, and created a plan for parties (page 55). A big key to my success was introducing other ways to relax during my day so my post-work drink wasn't so important to me. Becoming aware of my unconscious habit and making a few small changes reduced my calorie intake by about 150 empty calories a day. I can report that my beer belly shrank quite a bit (about 1 pound per month) for a while until I hit a plateau.

Comfort Without Food

If you can start managing some of the tension in your day using something other than food, you will lose weight (seriously). Most of the comforting ideas outlined in this chapter derive from a simple concept: Take a break.

Take a break!

The first question I ask a stressed-out friend when he is about to lose it is "What have you done for yourself today?" I am not talking about a one-hour massage at a spa. I have been so tense from work obligations (like writing this book), I haven't stopped to go to the bathroom or drink a glass of water. Okay, how crazy is that? A teeny break will allow you to tune in to your body and wake you up to the fact that whatever is upsetting you is temporary.

Take a page from smokers and take a nonsmoking break. I've never been a smoker and we all know how bad it is for your health, but getting away from your desk or other chores for five or ten minutes is good for body and soul.

Of course, when possible, explore some longer forms of nonfood comfort as well.

The Exercise Break

The obvious activity choice for any break longer than three minutes is exercise. I know it is difficult. Who the heck wants to put on their gym clothes when they could have a cookie? But if exercise can be your answer to stress in place of food, you will do yourself a world of good.

The shift to exercise as a response to stress began for me after I had my children. I found myself hitting the cookies, scones, and double mochas hard *every* day because I couldn't handle the screaming and unpredictability of their moods and actions. Don't get me wrong, my children fill me with wonder, love, and joy and I can't imagine my life without them. But let's just say I found their toddler behavior challenging. I was lucky in that I had the support of a partner who is more patient and less emotional than I am. One day as my daughter lost it again and I felt the urge to eat yet another cookie, my husband walked in the door. I asked him to watch the children and I walked outside for thirty minutes, came back, and resumed my parenting duties without the cookie. On my walk I passed other homes. I looked at the twinkly lights in those houses and remembered that there were many other parents going through the same thing, and I calmed down.

Can I take a walk every time my kids stress me out? Of course not, but I would be in seriously great physical shape if I could. I have found that if I do an exercise DVD during the day, my response to my children's fighting, frustration, and socks on the floor at the front door is different than if I sat on my couch or office chair for hours.

The mental benefits of aerobic exercise have a neurochemical basis. Exercise reduces levels of cortisol, the stress hormone. Exercise also stimulates the production of endorphins that relieve stress and pain, just like food and heroin do (see the beginning of this chapter). There is good news here—you can get addicted to the effects of exercise, the same way you get addicted to the calm feelings that come from sugary, fatty food. In the chapter on exercise (page 77), I'll share how to begin to love exercise and get in shape.

Is it easier to spray Cheez Whiz into your mouth? Why yes, it is, and I am not telling you that your Cheez Whiz days are over, but you can mitigate the eating response to stress by trying exercise as a response to stress.

Vacations

According to a 2011 survey by Expedia, the average American worker earns fourteen days off per year, but takes only twelve of them. About a quarter of Americans don't have any vacation time at all because they work in hourly jobs that do not provide paid time off. (Do I feel like an idiot suggesting that you take a vacation even if you can't afford it? Yes, I do.)

On the other hand, you might want to review the potentially dire health consequences of not taking time off. Just take a look at the incidence of heart disease in vacationers versus non-vacationers. One research study found that men who were at high risk for coronary heart disease and who failed to take annual vacations were 32 *percent* more susceptible to dying from a heart attack than at-risk men who did take a break. Another study compared women who vacationed at least twice a year to those who took one every six years or less. Incredibly, the women who did not vacation annually were almost *eight times* more likely to develop coronary heart disease or have a heart attack. So, do you want to live, or die working?

If you're among the 75 percent of Americans who do have paid vacation time (and can afford to use it), you must take it. A real break from the stress of your world will make a difference in your perspective and help you reset. I took my last vacation too long ago. My children swam around a big pool and were so tired at night that they fell asleep when their heads hit the pillow. I smelled the sea air and listened to the wind in the palm trees; I sat by the pool, fruity tropical drink in hand, and read a book—so relaxed I could hardly move. Right now, when I want to replay that mental tape of the wind and heat, I can hear and feel it. The benefits of my tropical vacation (less expensive in the off season) have stayed with me for years because when times are stressful, I remember all the laughter, sunshine, and peace. All the responsibilities that I have on a daily basis (packing lunches, rushing to get out the door, working, driving to tap lessons) were gone and I could just sit back and enjoy my kids. Did I have trouble turning off? Yes. Did I worry about the financial consequences? Yes. But in the end, the time off was priceless for my health and my family.

Taking a week or two to visit the beach or other relaxing locale may not be feasible for you, but you *can* have mini breaks, and these are still valuable. Try a long weekend in a restful spot a couple of hours from your home. It is important to get away from

---

TOP TEN WAYS TO TAKE A BREAK RIGHT NOW

1. Breathe deeply.
2. Picture a relaxing place such as a beach with turquoise water and white sand.
3. Look at a photo of a person who relaxes you.
4. Make—and drink—your favorite hot tea, without doing anything else.
5. Give someone a hug (or cuddle a stuffed animal if you are at work).
6. Massage your neck (or have someone else massage it for you).
7. Smile for two minutes.
8. Close your eyes.
9. Listen to some calming music.
10. Take a walk around the block or around your office.

the piles of dishes, laundry, and phone calls. How about checking out a local park or museum, or grabbing a coffee in a new café with a juicy book?

A "teensy break" can happen every day after or before work. For me that would be reading a few pages of a book or magazine, sitting on my couch listening to music, or walking outside to see what's going on with the weather. The key to the "teensy break" is to stop doing the necessary and draw your attention to something pleasurable that will remind you that you work to live, not live to work.

Meditation

The nice thing about meditation is that it is inexpensive and you don't need to go anywhere special to do it. The downside is that it can be a lot harder than it sounds. "Connect your mind and body to the present and your worries will melt away," says the meditation practitioner. Guided, mantra, mindfulness, and transcendental are all different flavors of meditation. Then there are the movement-based meditation practices of yoga, tai chi, and qi gong. There are books, videos, and classes on all of these methods for people who want to give them a try.

I have tried a bunch of meditation methods and found that I like yoga the best. I bought a DVD called *A.M. and P.M. Yoga* featuring Rodney Yee for $12 when I saw it next to the checkout at Walgreens. My search for calm was solved by an impulse purchase at a drugstore and I didn't even buy anything mind altering. I can't sit still for long and yoga allows me to move while I try to calm my mind and focus on the moment. Something about the pain in my hamstrings as I try to touch my toes gets me to pay attention to my body.

This video works for me because all I have to do is pop the disc into my computer; I don't have to change into yoga pants or jockey for position in a crowded class. The practice on the video is only about ten minutes long, and is set to relaxing music on a beach in Hawaii.

Keep Trying New Things

There are people around you who never relax. And there are others who have very stressful lives who seem to float above it all. I worked for a short period of time for a top executive of a large company who arrived at work every morning at 6 a.m. If you got into the office early enough, you could hear the sounds of gongs coming from his office, smell incense burning, and see him in his socks. That was how he dealt with the stress of his job. You too can find something out there that will calm you down and make life more fun.

The Less Obvious Forms of Emotional Eating

Boredom Eating

Gosh, I just love folding laundry. I get it all folded and open my fridge to see what delicious treat is waiting for me because I am so bored. How many years of my life have I lost folding pants, shirts, and underwear? Argh.

How often you feel bored is an important measure of satisfaction in your life. If you can't generate excitement about anything in your life, you could be clinically depressed, and you need to get help. On the other hand, there are just boring things we do every day that are hard to get through. My list includes dishes, laundry, driving my children to yet another play date, and vacuuming. So dull! I absolutely have to do this stuff but I don't derive much pleasure from these repetitive activities. I put my favorite tunes on but I still would rather be doing something else.

Eating something will give you an instant hit of pleasure. So how can you get pleasure when you are bored without resorting to food?

First, I want you to put crime scene tape (okay, masking tape will do) around your refrigerator.

Why? Because so many of us live in spaces where we are constantly walking through the kitchen. I can see the refrigerator from my favorite chair because my kitchen is also a living space.

Now, ask yourself why you are bored. I don't want to sound like some old grumpy person, but we live in an age of constant stimulation. Just like my kids who are constantly begging for attention, we check our phones every minute to see who is texting us. Nobody texted? What am I missing? How about a cookie? We are so overstimulated that a few minutes of silence can feel unpleasant.

I blame the television situation comedy. In these shows, there is nonstop action: friends dropping by unannounced (who does that?), funny arguments, stolen kisses, and continual excitement. Life, of course, moves at a much different pace. Our roommates aren't all happy and fun, our kids aren't always amusing, and we only have time to hang out at Starbucks once a week, not every day. Our lives *are* boring when you compare them to what you see in the movies and on TV.

My approach for dealing with boredom is to close my eyes and picture something else that I want to do other than eat. It's taken a lot of effort to get to this place, but now I will grab my knitting, open a book, or take a walk before I open the fridge. It is good to occupy your hands with something so you feel engaged. I try to have magazines or newspapers ready to grab so I stay away from food; if you're crafty, having a project on hand is useful. I do not turn on the TV when I am bored because there are a ton of advertisements for food that entice me. Friends tell me I should get a TIVO or DVR.

When you want to eat because you are bored ask yourself, "What do I really need right now?" The answers can be as varied as "I need a new job" or "I need a nap." You need to recognize when you are filling a need with food that would be better filled with something else.

Instead of eating, take a walk, cuddle your kid (or your sweetie or a pet), paint your nails, or draw a picture. If that's not enough, try chewing gum or eating something low calorie and crunchy, like celery.

Happy Eating

Maybe you aren't stressed out, bored, or angry. How about when you are feeling good? "Happy hours" celebrate the end of the workday. Woo-hoo! I finished a whole day and now I get a treat with my buddies.

You are feeling great and you want to extend that feeling with food. The problem is that the food you choose for happy eating usually isn't the healthiest. Buffalo chicken wings, deep-fried mozzarella sticks, loaded potato skins, and other unbelievably fatty snacks are the mainstay of happy hour. Why? Salty snacks make you thirsty, and you inevitably order more beer.

At one of my former jobs, the company sponsored a Friday happy hour every week to promote teamwork. Honestly, I thought I was going to turn into a deep-fried potato skin. My method for dealing with the work-sanctioned party every week was to change jobs.

Your happy food has to change, just like your comfort food has to change. Check out page 51 for tips on how to handle celebrations.

Life-Altering Catastrophes

There are events in life that are so stressful that no amount of deep breathing is going to help you. Divorce, job loss, death, or other traumatic events can wreak havoc on any healthy eating plan you have worked hard to create. Why do you think people bring cheese-filled casseroles to wakes? Can you imagine someone showing up with a kale salad and a side of tofu? Oh yes, after I watched my dearest friend get put in the ground, I need a big pile of tofu.

I have received e-mails from readers who can't get control of their eating when these types of things happen. I always tell them to let go, experience the emotions that are consuming them, and eat comfort food. Find a way to get to the other side, and then deal with the extra pounds. Why be angry with yourself when you are dealing with so much already?

When a friend of mine in graduate school found out that her husband of seven years was a closet transvestite, she moved out of her house and for a few months started every day with a large margarita. This ended after she drove over her roommate's cat, but the point is that she is now fine. She apologized profusely and bought her roommate a new cat. Now she has a career and a new partner and starts her day with a cup of coffee.

When I lost my beloved aunt, I found myself unable to get out of bed. I didn't want to put my feet on the ground to start my day knowing she was gone, so I just lay there until one of my children jumped on me and I had to deal with their needs. At the end of the day, I would lie down as soon as I could get away to examine the lines in the ceiling again. I am happy to say that, months later, I started getting up without relying on a child as an alarm clock.

Take the time to love yourself, find ways to heal, and allow yourself to be a mess for a while. If dealing with a catastrophic life event includes cheesecake, Doritos, and beer, then so be it. You can get back to being healthy when the worst of your pain and sadness is over.

Feeding Your Soul

Food is essential for survival and some would say that faith is as well. Snack Girl is far from a spiritual advisor, but what I do know is that an unconditional loving presence, however you name it, is important to our well-being. You've got to take care of yourself. Your physical self needs healthy food and water, and your emotional self needs to be nurtured and nourished as well.

Some of us are lucky—our families and communities provide enough support that we can just focus on the love we get and give. Others have to look harder to find the key to believing their lives have meaning. How you find your meaning is a subject for a different book, probably not written by me. If your soul needs some TLC and you aren't sure where to find it, start a conversation with people whom you love and respect.

People who have a partner or children usually talk about how they love them and find joy in the relationships closest to them. My family is the reason I get up in the morning, and my connections to my community and friends fill me with hope, love, and joy. I believe in my family and community. Focusing on how I impact them by being the best person I can be is my meaning in life.

I could give advice like "Turn off the TV," "Take a walk in the woods," "Call a good friend and listen hard to what they have to say," "Find a religious faith to embrace," or "Play with your kids." But is that helpful? I'm not sure. How you determine what feeds you (other than food) is a lifelong project. My only piece of advice is to look for the unconditional love that exists around you in human form. Know that people love you and try to love them back. If you can find peace in a friend's smile, you are in good shape.

Exercise

Why Exercise? Can't I Just Sit Here?

Exercise is defined as a "bodily exertion for the sake of developing and maintaining physical fitness." Doesn't that sound awful? "Exertion" sounds like work, and we are already working all the time. Most of us don't think that exercise is as important to our life as, let's say, breathing. If you stop breathing right now (hold your breath for a minute and try it), you will die. But what if I told you that exercise is as necessary to our bodies' healthy functioning as breathing? You would say: I'm sitting on the couch reading this book and I'm still alive.

A scientific study of 416,175 Taiwanese adults found those who exercised just fifteen minutes a day—or ninety minutes a week—extended their life expectancy by *three years* compared with those who did no exercise. I know you want to be there for all the great things that could happen in those three years—to see your youngest grandchild graduate from college or take off for a cross-country trip after you've retired.

I had a beloved aunt who died of lung cancer at sixty-three. She was a smoker and I know if she had her life to do over again, she would never touch a cigarette so she could be here longer to enjoy her family and friends. I will never forget the force of her anger over dying too soon. Her unintended gift to me was that she woke me up to the fact that every day here is precious. The difference is that cigarette smoking is something you have to stop, while exercising is something you have to start. It was easy for my family to point at cigarettes as the source of her too-early death. I don't know how many of us will be on our deathbed wishing we had walked around the block a couple of times a day to stay alive a few more years.

It seems like every day there is another study that recognizes exercise as an important factor for preventing or treating disease. Let's choose just one common problem: Seventy percent of Americans at some point in their lives have back pain. Research has shown that Pilates is an excellent cure for back pain. Go to the doctor and he or she might give you a prescription for a pain medication or suggest that you consider surgery. In an ideal world, you'd get a "prescription" for Pilates and insurance would pay for it. Which would you rather have? I know, the surgery. No, you don't! You want to do exercises to strengthen your stomach and back muscles so you are out of pain forever versus expensive back surgery that may or may not work.

How about colon cancer? It's the third leading cancer killer for women in the United States behind lung and breast cancer. Many studies have consistently found that adults who increase their physical activity, either in intensity, duration, or frequency, can reduce their risk of developing colon cancer by 30 to 40 percent relative to those who are sedentary. Unfortunately, if you start exercising after you get colon cancer it is too late to get the benefits.

Pick a problem: Are you not sleeping? Anxious? Lethargic? No sex drive? You need to exercise! Many scientific studies across disciplines support the fact that exercise is as fundamental to helping our bodies function correctly as eating healthy food, but we don't treat it that way.

How many of us treat exercise as *essential* to our lives? Frankly, I have always treated exercise as "something I will get to when I have the time." I remember in high school actively avoiding my physical education classes because they were so boring. One of my friends, who is now a physical trainer, used to sit outside her high school and smoke a cigarette instead of going to gym class. I'm not blaming our public education system for our collective lack of enthusiasm, but it seems to me that most of us felt we would be just fine without it.

Many of us are paying for gym memberships that we are not using because we can't find the time to do a workout. Why? Because we are too tired from managing our hectic lives to make time for ourselves. The irony is that we are exhausted precisely because we aren't taking care of the essentials for living well—healthy eating and exercise.

The Twenty-First-Century Challenge of Exercise

Sir Isaac Newton, an English physicist, stated in his first law of motion:

An object at rest stays at rest and an object in motion stays in motion.

It seems like everything around us encourages inactivity. As a society, we have done an incredible job of outsourcing any physical labor to machines that make life easy.

In the 1940s in my neighborhood in Amherst, Massachusetts, children walked to the two-room schoolhouse. I have talked with women in their eighties who lived this active life and are grateful for central heating and insulation, but they wax lyrical about ice skating for fun and (get this) country dances. People would chop wood to keep their houses warm. Everybody was a gardener whether they liked it or not; they needed the vegetables. Needless to say there was no 24 Hour Fitness franchise needed.

Our culture has made "movement" difficult to incorporate into our daily life. We have to plan for something our ancestors couldn't avoid. We have transformed exercise into a scheduled activity instead of an integral part of our lives. The irony—now that we have machines to perform boring physical labor, is that we need new machines to provide (some would say boring) physical exercise: treadmills, weight machines, and Nintendo Wii's. No one needed these machines or gym memberships back in the 1940s because everyone was moving all the time.

Forget going to the gym for a moment and ask yourself, "How much did I move today?" Did you walk to work or the train station? Or did you do what so many Americans do every day? Get in car, park as close to the office entrance as possible, sit at desk, drive home, sit on couch and watch television. The next question is, "How do you feel after a day like this?" If the answer is "like crap," join the club. Anything you could have done today to add movement would have made you feel a bit better. For example, you could have sat on a stability ball in front of the television instead of slumping on your couch. The ball is fun to sit on and keeps your muscles engaged while you sit burning calories and strengthening your core.

My Butt Was Glued to the Couch

I stopped moving when I had my children. All of a sudden, there were dents in the couch where butt cheeks had rested for many hours. In my defense, I was breastfeeding my first baby and my couch is very comfortable. At a certain point, I knew I had to get moving but I had no idea how to start. I lived in a big city, so I had a certain amount of pushing a stroller around, but that wasn't doing it for me. What I noticed is how I lacked energy and I didn't really *want* to move. I was stuck in a cycle of sitting, driving, sitting, nursing, and sleeping.

What may seem counterintuitive about adding exercise to your day is that it gives you energy even though it takes energy to do. I felt way too tired from sitting on my expanding rear to exercise, and I was not alone. Twenty-five percent of the general population experiences fatigue during the day. A University of Georgia study using sedentary individuals showed that a thirty-minute session three times a week of light cycling on a stationary bike can increase energy levels by 20 percent and decrease feelings of fatigue by 65 percent. The participants didn't even break a sweat on the test bike. How much would you give to feel energetic during the day instead of exhausted? No drug or energy drink on the market is going to touch a 65 percent decrease in fatigue.

A Five-Minute Action Plan

Do you have a comfortable pair of shoes and five minutes to spare? That's what got me moving when I couldn't conceive of what it would take to get me in any sort of shape where I felt good again. I took a personal trainer's advice and found just five minutes in my day to walk.

I put on my watch and walked for two and a half minutes away from my house and then two and a half minutes back. I committed to doing this every other day for a week. It felt so lame, but I just went ahead and did it. The next week I committed to ten minutes—five away and five back. The third week of walking I was up to fifteen minutes. And then I noticed something profound—*I felt like walking!*

If you had asked me before I started my first five-minute walk, "Do you want to walk today?" I would have said, "No way, I want to sit on this couch and turn on the boob tube." After a couple of weeks of doing just a little bit of exercise, I felt like getting off the couch. More importantly, if I took a day off from my walk—I missed it.

I didn't have $70 a month for a gym, and I didn't have an hour a day to exercise there anyway. I did have shoes and five to fifteen minutes per day. When I posted about my five-minute exercise regime on Snack Girl, I received a bunch of messages of support. April shared:

> *I started the same way in the fall of 2007. Just a few minutes around my apartment complex was all I could manage. After a few weeks my body could do more, but more importantly I WANTED to do more. Soon it wasn't 10–15 minutes 3 times a week; it was an hour 6 times a week. By the summer of 2009, I had dropped 100 lbs. I went from a size 18–20 to a size 4. All it took was commitment to it, which, once you get started, will be easy. You really do crave more once you get yourself going.*

Why did this work for April and me? We both set an achievable goal for starting exercise. Our goals fit our schedules, our fitness levels, and our budgets. We didn't attempt an hour of running because we were being kind to ourselves. Making that simple goal was enough to motivate us to the next level and give us momentum. My advice is to "set goal, achieve it, and repeat" until you are where you want to be.

I know it sounds nuts, but if you put this book down right now and take a little walk, you could start your future as a marathoner.

Don't Have Five Minutes? Try This

If I had my own action figure it would be the egg-shaped Weeble. Do you remember "Weebles wobble, but they don't fall down"? I sit in one place as much as I can and the top of me moves a little bit. The force of gravity on me, the desire to rest, seems integral to my being. For example, I took my son roller-skating at an indoor rink because it was raining. Did I roller-skate? No, I sat there and read O, *The Oprah Magazine* while he got a three-hour workout. I chose to *read* about self-improvement instead of actually improving myself. My kids love to sled when it is snowy and our yard isn't hilly, so I take them to their favorite sledding hill. Did I get out of the car and sled? No, I sat in the car and read *The New Yorker.*

Now, roller-skating and sledding are not my favorite things to do, but I need to exercise and in both instances I passed up my chance to move (and play with my kids) because of my internal gravity suck. I have outsourced exercise to "when I have time to go to the gym" instead of moving when I have the chance. Did I need to roller-skate for three hours or climb up the sledding hill until I was a sweating, sobbing mess? No, but I could have done something instead of nothing.

Let's say that committing to five minutes of walking will not work for you. What are your options? Add a bit of movement to your day and don't you dare call it exercise. Stop labeling "exercise" as this boring, painful activity that you must endure, and find opportunities to do something, whatever it is. I'm not talking about crazy stuff like squats while you brush your teeth. I am talking about super easy activities like walking to the farthest bathroom when you have to go.

Making movement a habit in your day will go a long way toward getting you in shape and will boost your energy level. I know it is hard to believe, but little steps are incredibly better for you than none at all. There are a couple of ways that I have added movement in my schedule without a big production:

1. Walk from the far end of the parking lot to the store I am visiting.

2. Carry my groceries to the car instead of pushing the cart when possible.

3. Sit on an inexpensive stability ball instead of the couch and keep my muscles engaged while reading or watching TV.

4. Mow my lawn, shovel the snow, bring in wood for the fireplace, carry out the trash, and vacuum the carpet.

You can also walk when chatting on the phone (both inside and outside) and listen to books while walking instead of sitting. You do not need a gym membership, a buddy, a pedometer, or a Nintendo Wii to get fit. You do need to start moving.

Use the Buddy System

Do you remember elementary school field trips? I remember getting assigned a buddy and hoping it wasn't the kid who picked his nose all day. The chaperones designed the buddy system so that we would look after one another. They didn't want anyone to get lost and miss the bus back to school.

When I first started my five-minute walks, I announced to one of my pals that I was trying to turn over a new leaf. Guess what? Susie was right there with me. Her desk job was taking its toll on her fitness level and she wanted to walk during her lunch hour. We had talked about having lunch together, but this was much better because we weren't spending money on Chinese takeout. One of the best parts of our weekly one-hour walk was that she worked next to San Francisco Bay and a wonderful paved trail. We saw birds, boats, and planes and got to talk about our personal challenges. She always pushed me to walk faster (nicely, of course) and I found myself looking forward to exercise.

We adults are lost without our buddies, too. It's estimated that up to 45 percent of fitness-club members quit going in any given year. Maybe we signed up for a whole year because of a post–New Year's sale. By March we have the guilt of having quit in February, and we're still paying the bills. Going it alone has its risks; the biggest is that you won't hold yourself accountable.

How to find a buddy isn't always obvious. One of my readers started posting about her workout ambitions and schedule on Facebook and a friend asked if she could join. Some entrepreneurial people start blogs (ahem) recording their progress to share it with family and friends. Though their buddies aren't with them on their workouts, they do provide support and encouragement with comments. You can set up a personal blog for free on Wordpress.com, which is incredibly easy to use. There is even a *Wordpress for Dummies* book if you are completely technically illiterate.

THE ARMS THAT INSPIRED A NATION

In 2008, a new first family moved into the White House. The First Lady dressed in sleeveless dresses that showed us a pair of fully toned arms with defined biceps and triceps. A whole nation of women went, "OMG, how do I get arms like that?"

I examined my own arms at that time and realized I had something called "bat wings." When I held up my arm a bit of flab would hang down, and that was not attractive. This part of my body had never bothered me until I took a hard look at Michelle Obama. She knew that the part of your body that everyone sees naked is your arms (unless you work as a swimsuit model).

Michelle Obama inspired me. I wanted *more* than to get moving. I wanted to transform my "bat wings" into a pair of "I can do ten real push-ups" arms. These arms would be shown off during the summer months when I wear my Target designer tank tops. Yes, I was going to be one hot mama, hanging out with my kids next to the Slip-N-Slide.

If there is absolutely no one who can be your buddy, use the staff at the gym. At the end of your treadmill session, before you walk out to your car, turn to the staff behind the desk and say, "See you tomorrow." When you arrive the next day, be sure to say hello. Repeat. This works great if you learn the staff's names. All of a sudden "Courtney at the gym" is your buddy! They will notice you and then, when you skip a day, you will hear, "Hey, where were you yesterday?" Yes! You have found someone to look after you.

There is another benefit to finding a pal to work out with you. Once you begin a regimen with one person, you might get lucky and find a whole bunch of people who are exercise hobbyists. This happened for me this year when I finally joined a women-only gym that didn't cost an arm and a leg. After going a couple of times on my own, I began to see women I knew from my various other "sitting down" activities. When I picked my kids up from school, a friend asked me when I was going to the gym. When I dropped off my office rent check, the assistant asked me about my favorite exercise classes. All of a sudden, my community began supporting me in my desire to get fit, and I hadn't even asked.

We all have communities that we involve ourselves in outside of work or the home. Maybe your church, book group, sports bar, or knitting circle is where you hang out. Now, if you are lucky, you can add friends who exercise to your community. Why is this great? Because you socialize with exercise as the focus versus food, knitting, watching sports, or other sedentary activities. You encourage each other just by talking about your goals, workouts, athletic gear, and favorite athletic trainers. We are in it together and instead of meeting for a drink after work, we put on our sneakers and go for a walk (and then maybe get the drink).

I'm Working Out but I'm Not Getting Fit

I have heard from my readers that the exercise they are doing isn't getting them the results they want. Why not? I have two theories on why we can't get in shape. First, we use food as a reward for exercise and, second, we avoid pain.

Food as a Reward

I believe we vastly overestimate the number of calories we can add to our diet because we are exercising. "I can have that cupcake because I did my walk today." I used to do this all the time. At the top of the hill I lived on in San Francisco was an adorable café that made irresistible peanut butter chocolate chip cookies. If I walked up this very steep hill, rather than driving, then I could have a cookie. I think I gained a couple of pounds with this strategy.

The average-size cupcake has 300 to 350 calories. A 155-pound person burns about 186 calories walking two miles in twenty-six minutes. The math is simple: Eat the cupcake, take the walk, and you're still taking in more calories than you're using. Weight Watchers gives you extra "activity points" to add to your daily total when you exercise. These points are helpful because you get to eat more, but I wonder if members start to see food as a reward for exercise. I do think it is important to realize that you are going to be hungrier when you start exercising more. The question is how you satisfy the hunger. Exercising more will, hopefully, inspire you to eat healthier. Now you get to eat more healthy food, hooray!

CALORIES IN TOP TREATS

Bakery cupcake	585
Glazed doughnut	200
Chocolate chip cookie	220
½ cup of Ben & Jerry's ice cream	260
12-ounce Starbucks Caffe Mocha	270

CALORIES BURNED BY A 155-POUND PERSON IN 30 MINUTES OF EXERCISE

Weight lifting	112
Walking at 3.5 mph	149
Hatha yoga	149
Disco dancing	205
Running at 5 mph	298

If you like to reward yourself for adding thirty minutes of exercise to your day, what should you give yourself? How about a new pair of cute underwear or some fresh flowers? For me, it would be ten minutes with my bedroom door closed and absolutely no one bothering me. Sometimes I hide in the bathroom to get time to myself (don't tell anyone). You could put a dollar in a jar every time you complete your workout and save up for a massage or a new pair of dope running shoes. Once you realize rewarding yourself for exercise with indulgent food is self-defeating, you can start to get creative about what else will work for you.

Don't Love Pain?

Do you ever see people running on the side of the road, looking great, and wonder how they do it? You know the type I am talking about. They are athletes who do 5Ks, marathons, triathlons, and mountain bike races on the weekends. They are fit.

Then, there are professional athletes. These people train to be the best at a sport and they awe us with their amazing feats. In his best-selling autobiography *Open*, Andre Agassi, one of my favorite pro athletes, describes his journey to professional tennis player; it is filled with physical pain. In a passage from the beginning of the book he describes the walk back to the locker room after winning an important match:

I hurry off the court. I don't dare stop. Must keep moving. I stagger through the tunnel, my bag slung over my left shoulder, feeling as if it's slung over

my right shoulder, because my whole body is twisted. By the time I reach the locker room I'm unable to walk. I'm unable to stand. I'm sinking to the floor. I'm on the ground . . . . I can't—I can't—breathe.

Agassi did this to himself. His tolerance for this kind of punishment is a big part of why he won eight grand slams.

Since I doubt anyone reading this book is planning to try to win one grand slam (forget eight), why do I bring this up? It has to do with what it takes to get in shape. How long can you be physically uncomfortable? When you stub your toe, do you scream for a medic? Do you give up the minute you start to perspire?

My action figure, the Weeble, doesn't like to hurt. She hates sweating and feeling like she can't catch her breath. When the going gets rough, she looks for a way to exit the room without anyone noticing.

On the other hand, I wanted those Michelle Obama arms. I wanted to feel as if I can lift my luggage into the overhead compartment on a plane without looking like I'm struggling. "No, sir, I can do it," I say confidently as I thrust the bag over my head like it weighs no more than a feather. I wanted to hike up the small hills around my house without craving an oxygen tank. To achieve these goals, I had to get uncomfortable.

The first indication that getting in shape was going to be harder than I thought was when I purchased one of the best-selling exercise DVDs on the market, *30 Day Shred* by Jillian Michaels. She says things like, "There is no modification for a jumping jack. I have four-hundred-pound people who can do a jumping jack and so can you." Right. I can do jumping jacks. "I am forty years old and I absolutely hate jumping jacks, but I am going to try," I told myself. After a few jumping jacks, my right ankle protested, and I modified my jumping jack with a step-touch move (enter the Weeble).

I could get through only ten of the twenty minutes of *30 Day Shred* when I first attempted it. I had trouble with *everything*: the push-ups, bicep curls, squats, jogging, and stretching. The day after my first attempt at the workout, I felt like I'd been hit by a truck. My arms burned, my gluteus maximus protested, and I felt like my teeth hurt. From a mere ten minutes of intense exercise, I was walking around moaning.

But I recognized that the pain was part of the process. I had to get uncomfortable if I wanted those arms and I could not avoid it. I hated it but I kept going.

After two months of attempting the workout a couple of times a week, I found that I could finish it. Jillian and Michelle inspired me to keep going. I was sweating within five minutes of starting the DVD and I started to get used to it. After a while, the bicep curls with my three-pound weights and modified push-ups felt easier and I started to see results.

What I learned is that you cannot fear pain. There will be pain. There will be fatigue. There will be moaning. But your body will start to feel alive. Like you plugged electrodes into your thumbs and big toes and attached your body to a battery. You will feel like a shot of energy has been zapped into you. Parts of you that have been sleeping will start to wake up (I think you know which parts I am referring to). There is a fine line between pain and pleasure, and you will cross it many times.

> **FAVORITE WORKOUT DVDS**
>
> Jillian Michaels: *30 Day Shred*
> New York City Ballet: *Workout*
> Rodney Yee: *Power Yoga Collection*
> Jillian Michaels: *Ripped in 30*
> *The Biggest Loser: The Workout—Boot Camp* with Bob Harper

The nice thing about exercise DVDs or online classes is that they are relatively inexpensive—sometimes free in the case of online videos—and you can use them as suits your schedule. The downside is that no one is holding you accountable. When I told a friend about my exercise DVD collection, she told me she loved to watch them sitting on her couch.

I'm Ready to Get in Shape: What Should I Do?

I'm a big believer in not thinking too hard before you start a new project. When it comes to choosing the best type of exercise, I take the spaghetti-on-the-wall approach: Throw a whole bunch of things out there and see what sticks.

For example, I noticed a new gym on my way home from work and called to ask about the prices and facilities. They wouldn't quote me a price on the phone and asked me to make an appointment. I did, and they wanted me to sign up for three sessions a week with a trainer, at $65 each. For the low price of $780 per month, I could get in shape. I went home and told my husband we needed to take out a loan. Just kidding! I thanked the woman for her time, got into my 1984

Honda (worth less than one month at that gym), and drove home. This was not my solution.

Next! After reading about people who could walk on a treadmill and type on their computer, I decided to design my own desk. I bought a used treadmill on Craigslist and put it in my office. I managed to hook up my computer so I could walk and type at the same time. It became obvious after I fell off a couple of times that, while a great idea for some people, the "treadmill desk" was an absolute failure for me. I gave up and sold the treadmill on Craigslist before its presence depressed me.

I have tried step aerobics (hated them), hot yoga (oy!), and ankle weights (torturous). I have also tried spinning, weight machines, and Pilates and I love them all. Helping Americans get in shape is big business, and I think that is good news. Even in my small town, there are Zumba classes, a rock-climbing gym, and an ice-skating rink.

You have to believe that something is going to work for you. I keep trying stuff because I am one of those people who get bored easily. If going to the next fitness class seems like a burden, then I won't go. So, I try to mix it up. My latest obsession, which will probably be over by the time you are holding this book, is "boot camp." Whoever designed boot camp was trying to kill me. I have been at the point of tossing my cookies many times in this class, and yet, for the last two months, I keep going back. My teacher switches the activity every minute or so, until you fall down (not really). Why do I keep going back? Because at the end of the class I feel so great, like I've been locked in a hotel room with my husband for a couple of days. Yes, the rush of endorphins, or feel-good hormones, is intoxicating.

What about the arms? I found that the key to having cut arms is to work my biceps and triceps.

TEN GROUP EXERCISE CLASSES TO TRY

1. Zumba—Latin American dance workout
2. Spinning—stationary bike workout
3. Power yoga—strength and stretching
4. Pilates—core strengthening based on training for ballet
5. Boot camp—military style circuit training
6. Kick boxing—kick and punch for a cardio workout
7. Tai chi—martial arts for strength and agility
8. Aerobics—low-impact or high-impact movement
9. Aqua fitness—exercise in water, low impact on joints
10. Hip hop—dance moves for fitness

After only a month of hitting them once a week with simple curls, my "bat wings" shrank quite a bit. It amazed me how a little bit of effort could make such a difference.

Get Thyself a Routine

When you have a crazy day that falls down around you, what do you do? Do you walk in the door at 6 p.m. and grab your sneakers, ready to start your walk, or do you sit your butt on your couch? Most of us pick the couch because we are so overwhelmed we just need to stop.

Much of the time, we put ourselves after our jobs, spouses, children, or whatever is right in front of us demanding our attention. The short-term result is that we are proud that we helped out, but the long-term result will cost you.

One of my best buddies, a Harvard MBA, was thrilled to have become a president of a division of a large company. I saw him when he started the job and he was giddy with excitement. About four months later, I saw him again and he looked completely different. His BlackBerry was beeping all the time and his face was twisted with frustration. His partner told me that he hadn't stopped working for a day since the job began. At the ripe old age of forty, he ended up in the emergency room with chest pains. The whole story sounds like a cliché because it is. Every day, he managed to let the insanity of his day affect his health until his body told him to stop it.

Say it out loud: *I will not sacrifice my health for the potential craziness of my day.*

Now that we have agreed that you will take care of yourself, how do you do it? Many exercise first thing, before anything can interfere. On *60 Minutes*, Martha Stewart was interviewed on her treadmill at 4:30 a.m. before her day began. The CEO of a media corporation, she didn't even allow a major network news show to stop her exercise routine. I like that kind of grit and we all need to get some.

Some ideas to help you begin your day with exercise are going to bed earlier so you are ready to get up earlier, sleeping in your athletic clothes, and having a partner who wakes you up and encourages you. Personally, I have never been able to get up like Martha and exercise. I have tried it and I always feel like I am going to die at 5 a.m.

The "after work" exercisers, like my Harvard MBA buddy, have more of a challenge. My favorite solutions include not sitting down when you come home, putting your sneakers in front of your door so you change into them before you even walk into your house or apartment, and lugging your gym bag everywhere. Do not give yourself an excuse to stop moving. Remember the object that stays at rest?

You have to make exercising a habit that is nonnegotiable. If you are tired, you will start to bargain with yourself and get out of any hard work that's part of your day. You are only hurting yourself when you allow life to get in the way. You must:

- Find fun ways to incorporate movement into your daily life.
- Not give up when a new exercise regime doesn't work for you.
- Believe that the more exercise you do, the more you will want to do.
- Not fear pain; endure it and you will be rewarded.
- Not allow crazy days to get in the way.
- Begin to see exercise as a gift to yourself rather than a burden.

Your whole life could change if you develop a great exercise habit.

Food Marketing

Where's the Juice?

The inspiration for Snack Girl started with a purchase in a San Francisco café. I was hanging out with my two-year-old daughter and wanted to get her a special drink. There was an open cooler at her height and she picked out a Snapple with drawings of pineapple and strawberries and the words "All Natural" displayed across the front. Assuming it was 100 percent juice, I happily purchased it for her, grabbed my coffee, and sat down. As I reported in the Introduction, I read the label and was shocked to find out that her drink contained high-fructose corn syrup, artificial colors, artificial flavors, and only a small percentage of juice. Honestly, I had no idea what I was buying for my daughter and I felt angry.

Before having a baby, I would drive like a maniac. After having a baby, I drove as if my car were covered in bubble wrap and I started to make full stops at stop signs. Before Ruby, I glanced at the front of a food package, tossed it in my cart, and thought I was doing a good job feeding myself and my husband. Now, I check the back of the package to evaluate the ingredients and the nutrition facts. Yes, having children woke me up to the fact that I had no idea what I was buying most of the time.

There is one way to never be tricked about what you are buying: Don't buy any processed food. Stick to fresh fruits and vegetables. Buy oranges and a juicer. Make your own bread, yogurt, and cereal. Buy lots of glass Mason jars and fill them with nuts, whole grains, and dried beans. Get a canning kit and buy cases of fresh tomatoes. Start a kitchen garden. Your pantry will begin to be unrecognizable to most American households and you will strike fear in the hearts of executives of General Mills, Unilever, and Nestlé. The further you stay away from packaged food, the less time you have to spend reading labels.

I applaud people who are able to avoid processed food completely and I have attempted to do so myself. The problem is that processed food is convenient and I am busy. I want and need shortcuts. For example, if my children's school is having a bake sale for a fund-raiser, do I get out my mixer and bake homemade cupcakes, or do I use a cake mix and save myself thirty minutes of prep time and cleanup? I use the cake mix, but I do alter it to make it a little healthier (page 262). When there is a birthday in our family, however, the choice is obvious. I ask my husband to bake a cake and demand butter cream icing.

My product choices are the result of learning the marketing tricks and ingredients of the food industry. I have gotten to be an expert on figuring out which products are decent and which are healthy fakes, junk food, or too high in fat, sodium, or sugar to be a truly healthy choice. Along the way, I have consulted with registered dieticians and toured grocery stores with them to find the most nutritious choices. This chapter is a summary of what I have learned to help you breeze through the supermarket knowing you have done the best for yourself and your family.

The Images on Food Packages

Do you remember "generic food"? Back in the seventies, many stores had an aisle of white packages with black letters spelling out what was inside. I remember boxes of corn flakes and cans labeled simply "peas," "corn," and "chicken soup"—no beautiful photographs or graphics, no banner copy declaring "Improved" or "All Natural." Now imagine an entire store with those white packages and ask yourself how you would choose which one to buy. Obviously, you would read the nutrition facts and ingredients list to find out what was in the product.

Frequently, we choose something based on the pictures on the package, as I did with the Snapple. Why would those images be misleading? Food manufacturers are not in the business of honesty; they are trying to sell food. Their agenda is making money because they are beholden to their shareholders and owners. I'm not a conspiracy theorist, but it helps to remember that your best interest (eating less and healthier) and food companies' interest (making money) are at odds most of the time. A ton of marketing money has been spent on finding out what images and words appeal to consumers. In the United States, the Food and Drug Administration (FDA) is tasked with keeping food companies from printing flagrant lies on the package.

At a nutrition conference, I got a chance to question a high-ranking official at the FDA about why food packages are deceptive. I asked her about a famous brand of toaster pastries that is covered in beautiful photos of blueberries. There are no actual blueberries in the pastry! The brand lists only "blueberry extract" in the ingredients on the back of the package. The official told me that the agency receives a ton of complaints about packages like the one I described, and explained that under the First Amendment, companies are guaranteed a right to free speech. Unless they lie outright on their package, the FDA can't make them change it. So we are stuck with packages covered in blueberries when the reality is that the product is mostly flour and sugar with a little blueberry extract thrown in.

The Words on Food Packaging

Not only are we misled by the images on packages, but we're also attracted to phrases that confirm those images. One of my favorite examples is a packaged fruit snack, which parents buy because it is "made with real fruit." How badly do we want to believe that these cute little bags of gelatin and fruit juice are healthy for our kids? Our kids love them, and the term "real fruit" allows us to justify purchasing them, even though they are basically a form of candy.

The words and phrases that work on us are usually related to the latest food fad. So many of the buzz terms are about what the product lacks. Isn't that funny? Food marketers trumpet their products as "zero" this and "low" that. Wouldn't it be great if they told us what the product *does* have? Many of these phrases are pretty silly when you know something about food. For example, a brand of tortilla chips that have always been made with just corn, oil, and salt now advertises they are "whole grain" and "gluten free" on the front of the package. Nothing about them is different: The manufacturer has simply changed how it markets the chips because it knows that right now people are focused on adding whole grains to their diet and avoiding gluten. Are they healthier for you? Nope, they are still highly processed chips.

The images and phrases on most food packages may not be outright lies, but they are frequently deceptive. Decide you will ignore all of it and arm yourself with the knowledge on the nutrition label to evaluate the products you buy.

Good Processing Versus Bad Processing

Food processing is the transformation of raw ingredients into some other form. Obviously, there are some foods that you don't have to process to eat, like apples. We process food all the time when we cook at home. If I make a stir-fry, I "process" the vegetables by chopping them and sautéing them in a wok.

However, another kind of processing that we all know is more sinister. "Eatertainment" is a noun that I made up to define this phenomenon. The most obvious forms of eatertainment are prizes found in cereal boxes and Happy Meals at McDonald's. My children will say they are hungry just to get a toy.

There are more subtle forms of eatertainment. For example, I would argue that it is more fun to pick up a chicken nugget and dip it in sauce than gnaw on a chicken leg. How about Cheetos? Would you rather eat some cheese and crackers or chomp into a brightly colored puff of cheesy, salty flavor? Eatertainment is everywhere you

---

10 FOOD BUZZ WORDS AND PHRASES

1. Organic
2. Gluten free
3. Real
4. All natural
5. Reduced sodium
6. Low fat
7. Whole grain
8. Zero grams of trans fat
9. High fiber
10. No added sugar

look and I cannot argue that serving a football-shaped ice cream cake at a Super Bowl party isn't fun.

Start to look at your favorite foods and ask yourself if you are eating them because they are healthy or they are eatertainment. I bet the eatertainment foods are the most processed junk in your diet. An apple can't hold a candle to a bag of Doritos when it comes to fun. The brightness of the package, the smell, and the blast of flavor that comes from these chips are all notoriously addictive. But the Doritos have over thirty-three ingredients, including 220 grams of sodium in a one-ounce portion (and when was the last time you ate one ounce of Doritos?) and almost zero nutrition.

Have I come to the conclusion that all food processing is bad? Absolutely not. For example, I love frozen chopped vegetables. Frozen vegetables are less expensive than their fresh counterparts, are almost (and sometimes more) nutritious than fresh, and are great when I don't have time to do a lot of dinner prep. Many of the recipes in this book feature them because they are so easy to use (for example, Beef and Veggie Cottage Pie, page 178).

How about canned vegetables, like tomatoes? There has been concern over the toxicity of a chemical, BPA (bisphenol A), that has been used in the lining of cans to prevent corrosion. However, major manufacturers are phasing out its use and you can now find BPA-free cans on supermarket shelves. In my opinion, using canned vegetables or fruits (without large amounts of salt or sugar added) is another great shortcut.

Finally, there are companies that make products without chemical additives or preservatives. I would love to be able to name "brands you can trust" right here and say, "Buy these without question." But I have watched some of my favorite brands get purchased by larger companies, and then change the types and formulation of their products. For example, Kashi, a cracker and cereal brand founded in 1984, was purchased in 2000 by Kellogg's. Kashi is famous for using seven different whole grains in its food products. Kashi does use whole grains, but it also uses white flour (not whole wheat) to make its crackers, cereal bars, and some cereals. So, its products aren't 100 percent whole grain. The problem is that Kashi's "seven whole grains on a mission" marketing gives the impression that all the brand's products are whole grain, and many of them are not. Is this Kellogg's influence? I don't know. Kashi says it is run independently, but if a big cereal company owns you, don't they have some say in how you run your company? I find it hard to believe Kellogg's isn't advising Kashi on how to make profitable granola bars, cereals, and crackers.

Cost and Processing

It is a cold hard fact that processed foods made with wholesome ingredients, less sugar and sodium, and fewer additives cost more than their less expensive counterparts.

Why would *more* processing mean the product costs *less*? A great example is granola bars. A Quaker chewy granola bar costs less than half the price of a KIND bar. Why? Quaker's bar has forty-three ingredients, including corn syrup, partially hydrogenated soybean oil, and the preservatives BHT and TBHQ. The KIND bar has no preservatives and twelve ingredients, including dried fruit, whole grains, nuts, and sugar (non-GMO glucose and honey in the Almond and Apricot bar). Which do I buy? I cringe at the price and buy the KIND bar. It has much less added sugar, it tastes better, and it is more nutritious. I look at it as an investment in my health.

When we buy food, we tend to act like consumers looking for a great deal, but buying food shouldn't be treated the same as "where can I get the best price for a flatscreen television." Give yourself the gift of quality food products. You deserve the best you can afford when you pick out food for your family.

How to Evaluate the Nutrition Facts Label

Ingredients

The first step to choosing healthier packaged food is to imagine the box or can without the beautiful images. Spin the package around and read the first ingredient and you will immediately be able to judge what is the largest component of the food product.

Food manufacturers are required to list all of the ingredients in the product on the label in order of amount, from largest to smallest. For example, in my recipe for chocolate chip cookies, I use more flour than any other ingredient, so my ingredient list would start with flour. Sugar, butter, eggs, chocolate chips, baking powder, and vanilla follow in descending order.

I know that people are freaked out about food additives such as ammonium sulfate, red #5, or monosodium glutamate, and you can find these nonfood-sounding ingredients at the end of many lists. Most of these chemicals are used in small amounts to help with food preservation, color, and flavor. I'm not saying you shouldn't avoid them if they bother you, but I think they get more attention then they deserve. For me, the important information is right at the beginning of the list.

Take packaged bread. The front label may say "Made with whole grains," but if the ingredient list starts with "wheat flour," that indicates that whole grains are not the primary ingredient, even though some have been added. If the front label says "100 percent whole wheat" or the first words on the ingredient list are "whole-wheat flour," the product is all or mostly whole grain. One word—"whole"—makes a world of difference on the relative healthiness of the bread.

If you pick up a box of ice pops that says they are "made with real fruit" on the front of the box, check that ingredient list. There are wonderful pops that have pineapple or strawberries as the first ingredient. Then there are others whose ingredient list starts with sugar or high-fructose corn syrup. If you are looking for a healthier box of ice pops, buy the one that has actual fruit as the top ingredient. Remember, manufacturers can still cover their boxes with photos of strawberries even if they use only "strawberry extract."

Michael Pollan trumpeted the importance of the number of ingredients in his book *Food Rules*. His rule is that if the product has more than five ingredients, it should be avoided. Also, he promotes the idea that all ingredients should be recognizable, and we should avoid high-fructose corn syrup. You know, if you stick to these rules, you will be doing well. But they are general rules that have many exceptions, so I have developed my own product-specific guidelines (see page 102).

Nutrition Facts

The nutrition facts label is a gift to consumers, even though it lists a whole bunch of information that may or may not be relevant to how healthful a single food product is.

However, once you learn what information is important, you will be able to pick out "food fakes" like a superhero.

In 1990, President George H. W. Bush signed a law that required a nutrition label on packaged food regulated by the FDA. It took thirty-five different versions and lots of committees to come up with the label on all those packages. Do I think it is confusing? Yes, but I do think they tried to help us. The problem is that you have to be educated about how to use the information on the label, and most of us aren't.

Start at the beginning of the label and check out the serving size. I cannot tell you how many times I think what I am eating has 100 calories only to find out that I ate three servings and actually ingested 300 calories. For example, one brand of packaged bread lists one slice per serving and a different brand will have two slices per serving. Next look at the calories per serving.

The label then lists three nutrients you should try to limit: fat, cholesterol, and sodium. On the far right is the "percentage daily value" of these nutrients in the food. **Five percent or less is low** and you should feel good about purchasing the item. However, **20 percent or more is high,** and you need to be careful how much you consume. Then you'll see the micronutrients that you want to get enough of—for example, fiber, vitamin A, vitamin C, calcium, iron. Obviously, your goal is to get 100 percent of these per day. I always check these quickly in the hopes that I find a high number to support my colon, immune system, bones, or any other body function that could use some help.

It is a really good idea to familiarize yourself with the labels of the packaged foods you buy often. This knowledge will help you make

Nutrition Facts

Serving Size 1 cup (228g)
Servings Per Container about 2

Amount Per Serving

Calories 250	Calories from Fat 110

	% Daily Value*
Total Fat 12g	**18%**
Saturated Fat 3g	**15%**
Trans Fat 3g	
Cholesterol 30mg	**10%**
Sodium 470mg	**20%**
Total Carbohydrate 31g	**10%**
Dietary Fiber 0g	**0%**
Sugars 5g	
Proteins 5g	

Vitamin A	4%
Vitamin C	2%
Calcium	20%
Iron	4%

* Percent Daily Values are based on a 2,000 calorie diet. Your Daily Values may be higher or lower depending on your calorie needs:

	Calories:	2,000	2,500
Total Fat	Less than	65g	80g
Saturated Fat	Less than	20g	25g
Cholesterol	Less than	300mg	300mg
Sodium	Less than	2,400mg	2,400mg
Total Carbohydrate		300g	375g
Dietary Fiber		25g	30g

For educational purposes only. This label does not meet the labeling requirements described in 21 CFR 101.9.

informed choices throughout the day about what and how much you need to eat to be more or less healthy. Keep in mind that the best foods don't have a nutrition facts label at all (those are the ones that you don't have to worry about eating).

Evaluating Sweet Foods

The first number that I check out on any product in the sweet area of the flavor spectrum is grams of sugar. Five grams of sugar is about one teaspoon; picture that teaspoon when you read the label. Plenty of whole foods like grapes, milk, and red peppers contain natural sugar; my concern is the amount of sugar food manufacturers have *added* to the product. Since I love coffee, I imagine adding the listed grams or teaspoons of sugar to my coffee and decide whether I would drink it.

What foods surprise me with the amount of added sugar? Not Ben & Jerry's Cherry Garcia or Oreos. The ones that blow my mind are the ones that don't need any sugar (or only a wee bit) and end up with more per serving than a Coca-Cola (which has 39 grams of sugar in a 12-ounce can). For example, Mott's applesauce has 14 grams of *added* sugar in 4 ounces (or ½ cup). The total amount of sugar in a serving is 25 grams because apples have natural sugar. Applesauce is a perfectly reasonable processed food, but not when you kill its health benefits by cranking up the sugar. I buy unsweetened applesauce and have been known to make my own when I am deluged with apples in the fall.

There has been a big media frenzy over "hidden sugar" or sugar that has crept into healthy foods. Ketchup, salad dressing, and tomato sauce were flamed for having added sweeteners. Should sugar be added to these foods? Maybe a little, but the sugar problem isn't about condiments per se. The issue is the amount of added sugar consumed after a full day of eating processed foods. Personally, I don't think most added sugar has been hiding because it is in black and white in the nutrition facts portion of the box. We need to wake up and read the label so we know how much is there.

How much added sugar is too much? I have created rules for different foods (which I will cover in the next section), but I have noticed a marked difference in my tolerance for sugar as I have become healthier. Once you cut down on the doughnuts and increase the amount of fresh fruits and vegetables you eat, your taste for sugar will change. Processed foods that you used to crave start to taste too sweet. Yogurt is one of those foods that needs less and less sugar to taste good. My taste buds freaked out at the 18 grams of sugar (14 of them added) in a 5-ounce Chobani strawberry Greek yogurt. Keep eating healthy foods and you won't need to read the nutrition facts to know a product is loaded with added sugar.

Evaluating Savory Foods

It should come as no surprise that just as you need to review the grams of sugar for sweet foods, so should you check the amount of sodium in savory foods. Too much sodium in your diet can increase your blood pressure and your risk for heart attack and stroke. Heart disease and stroke are the leading causes of death in the United States, possibly because most Americans consume 3,300 milligrams of sodium per day, which is twice the recommended amount for most adults.

You won't be surprised to hear that food manufacturers add a ton of salt so that foods taste good. Salt is cheap and the right amount (usually a lot) makes food taste better. If you buy canned soup or frozen meals, you can easily eat a day's worth of sodium in one serving. Campbell's Harvest Vegetable soup boasts 1,300 milligrams of sodium for two cups, or the entire bowl-shaped package. The serving size is supposed to be one cup, but most people would eat the whole 120-calorie bowl for lunch.

How much sodium is too much? The 2010 Dietary Guidelines for Americans state that adults should consume no more than 2,300 milligrams per day, and 1,500 milligrams if you are fifty-one and older. A teaspoon of salt has 2,300 milligrams of sodium, so you can see the problem. A McDonald's Big Mac has 970 milligrams of sodium. Add a large fries (350 milligrams) and you are almost done for the day if you are fifty-one. The minute you buy a frozen meal or eat out, you will have trouble staying under the daily recommended amount.

My strategy is to buy no-salt processed foods (soups or frozen meals) and then add my own salt if necessary. I do make my own soups (see page 159) because it's so easy. I have been slowly cutting my consumption of takeout, fast food, and pizza over the years. Recently, I was at a party where pizza was served and I found myself (almost) not able to eat it because it tasted like someone had drowned it in salt. Just as with sugar, you will become aware of the saturation of salt in your food when you stop eating processed meals.

Tips for Common Pantry Items

To make it easier for you to breeze through the grocery store, I have put together some tips that help me in my own hunt for better foods. These are guidelines, not absolutes. You can find exceptions to every food rule out there. My favorite exception to the "fewer than five ingredients is better for you" rule is Fritos, which have only three (corn, oil, salt): Fritos have 20 grams of fat and 320 milligrams of sodium in a 2-ounce serving.

Cereal, Granola Bars, and Cereal Bars

The cereal aisle is notorious for statements like "supports your immune system" on a package of Kellogg's Fruit Loops. Yeah, so Kellogg's added vitamin C to the cereal, but the first ingredient is sugar (12 grams per serving) and it also includes three artificial colors and partially hydrogenated vegetable oil. I asked a couple of my registered dietician pals about how they navigate this aisle and came up with this list:

THE DO-I-BUY-IT CEREAL TEST

1. **Is the first ingredient a whole grain?** If it isn't whole grain, then it's a refined grain, which lacks nutrients and fiber.

2. **Is the sugar per serving 5 grams or less?** You are going to add milk and possibly some fruit to your cereal. Milk has sugar in the form of lactose and fruit has fructose, so you want to start with a cereal that is low in sugar.

3. **Does one serving provide at least 4 grams of fiber?** The amount of fiber indicates whether the cereal is entirely whole grain or a mix of whole-grain and refined-grain ingredients.

Cereals that meet those requirements are hard to find. I once told my children that they could purchase any cereal that passed the test. After thirty minutes of looking, they gave up. Beware that some of the cereals that do pass, like Cheerios and Shredded Wheat, have variations with added sugar that fail the test, such as Honey Nut Cheerios (9 grams of sugar) and Frosted Mini-Wheats (11 grams of sugar).

I use this test for granola bars and cereal bars as well. It is extremely difficult to find a granola or cereal bar with 5 grams or less of sugar, so do not become discouraged. Evaluating the grams of sugar in these products will teach you which are more like cookies than breakfast. When buying granola bars that contain dried fruit, check for added sugar in the ingredient list. The DIY breakfast bar recipe (page 132) has more than 5 grams of sugar because of mashed bananas and dried fruit, not added sugar.

Eggs

Snack Girl has gotten a lot of questions about eggs. I happen to love eggs: scrambled, soft-boiled, sunny side up, in omelets, yum! They are a relatively cheap form of protein and they have 70 calories each. The American Heart Association says you can eat one egg yolk per day, so I try to keep to that number to keep my cholesterol in check as long as I limit cholesterol from other sources (meat, poultry, and dairy products). Egg whites don't contain cholesterol, so you don't have to worry about eating too many. Unfortunately, egg whites also don't contain many of the nutrients in eggs, so I still eat yolks.

> **CEREALS THAT PASS THE TEST**
>
> Post Grape-Nuts
>
> Kellogg's Mini-Wheats
>
> Weetabix
>
> Cheerios
> (exception: 3 grams of fiber)
>
> Uncle Sam Original Cereal
>
> Barbara's Bakery Original Puffins
>
> Kashi Heart to Heart

For example, an egg yolk has 21.9 milligrams of calcium; the white, only 2.3. There is zero vitamin A, D, E, or K in the white versus the yolk, which contains all of these vitamins in varying amounts.

Not only are there nutritional claims on egg cartons, but there may be terms such as "organic" and "cage free." "Organic" indicates that the chickens have been fed feed that was not grown with pesticides, and "cage free" refers to the treatment of the birds.

My favorite advice about eggs is in Marion Nestle's book *What to Eat*; she spends twenty-five pages talking about them, then summarizes:

From a nutritional standpoint, eggs are eggs. Turning eggs into a "designer" food is a great way to get you to pay more for them but there are less expensive and easier ways to get vitamin E, selenium, lutein, and omega-3's from foods.

I ignore all the nutritional and environmental claims and buy local eggs. If you can find eggs produced at a small farm near you, buy them; these will be the freshest, tastiest eggs. I have tried them all, and this is my solution to the egg dilemma. My local supermarket carries local eggs, so you don't necessarily have to go to a specialty store or farmer's market to find them. Ask the manager of your supermarket if he or she has a local egg brand and try it. You might fall in love (with the eggs, not the supermarket manager).

Bread, Crackers, and Tortillas

Whole-wheat flour, yeast, water, and a little bit of salt and sugar are all it takes to make bread. Leave out the yeast, roll out the dough, and cut it into shapes and you have crackers. Add some oil or lard and you have tortillas. Alas, these products cause me the most headaches because they have a bunch of preservatives, artificial sweeteners, added sugars, dough conditioners, and all kinds of stuff that sounds like it belongs in a science lab.

When you're buying packaged bread, the rules are much the same as for cereals. Even if the front of the package says "Made with Whole Grains," check the ingredients list to see whether the first ingredient is a whole grain, such as whole-wheat flour. Companies will add whole grain to their products, but what you want is *100 percent whole grain*. Also check to see if there are more than 4 grams of fiber per serving. That amount is a good indicator that the bread is 100 percent whole grain, but also can mean that they added fiber in the form of cellulose powder.

After you check for 100 percent whole grain, you need to look at both the sugar and sodium amounts, and whether they're for one slice or two.

If you are buying "light" bread, be aware that artificial sweeteners are frequently added to make the bread sweet while keeping the calorie count down. I purchased these cute little round breads for my kids without noticing the added sucralose. My advice is to find bread with a short list of ingredients that you recognize and control the portion size instead of eating "light" breads.

It's taken me years to find brands of packaged breads that meet all my requirements; see below. The Alvarado Bakery and Ezekiel breads can be found in my local supermarket in the natural foods freezer. I store these in my freezer and thaw slices as needed because they have no preservatives and tend to mold before I get a chance to eat the whole loaf. Are they expensive? Yes, they can cost more than your usual brands, but you are getting better ingredients, tastier bread, and less to worry about.

The healthier crackers in the list can be found on the bottom shelf of the cracker aisle. You really have to hunt to find them, but they are there if you look. If you are used to salty and buttery Ritz crackers, these crackers will shock you with their bland crunchiness. You add the flavor by topping them with cheese, peanut butter, or whatever you like. When you allow food manufacturers to add the flavor, they also add a bunch of artificial ingredients that you don't need.

I'm still searching for the perfect tortilla. I buy the 100 percent whole-wheat variety; I find them in the refrigerator case next to the cheese. These still have more sodium than I would like, so I always keep my eyes out for new brands.

> **WHOLE-GRAIN BREAD AND CRACKER BRANDS**
>
> Alvarado St. Bakery sprouted bread and tortillas
>
> Ezekiel 4:9 sprouted bread
>
> Whole Foods 100% whole-grain bread
>
> Doctor Kracker
>
> Mary's Gone Crackers
>
> Ryvita crackers
>
> Wasa crackers

Yogurt

Packaged yogurt has exploded in the dairy aisle with all sorts of different varieties, brands, and claims. The biggest issue with yogurt is the amount of sugar per serving in the fruit-added and flavored varieties. I have seen all brands of yogurt that aren't the 100-calorie variety include 18 to 20 grams of sugar for a 5-ounce serving. When you add 3 teaspoons of sugar (15 grams) to 5 ounces of *anything* it becomes a dessert.

The health benefits of yogurt—live cultures, calcium, protein—are mitigated by all that sugar.

Most of the 100-calorie yogurts contain artificial flavors and sweeteners. None of these taste very good to me, so I avoid them.

I buy my favorite brand of plain whole-milk (not low-fat) yogurt and add jam, honey, or granola myself. I choose to eat less of a full-fat variety than eat the low-fat or nonfat version because I dislike the texture and taste of yogurts without fat; if you like low- or nonfat yogurt, use it. I save money because I buy a 32-ounce container versus a bunch of small containers, and I save calories because I don't add a lot of sugar. If you have small Mason jars, it is fun to buy apricot, strawberry, and blueberry jams, mix them with the yogurt to make different flavors, and store them in the fridge for a grab-and-go snack. My kids love these!

Juice

One of the most deceptive products in the supermarket is juice. I can't tell you how many times I have been tricked by the packaging, and it infuriates me. There are basically two kinds of juice:

1. 100 percent fruit juice
2. A little bit of fruit juice with water, sugar, and all sorts of stuff added

Which do I buy? I try to buy 100 percent fruit juice because it has some of the vitamins and minerals from the fruit that was squeezed to make it. Is juice as good for you as eating the fruit? No—it has no fiber, and juice is a concentrated form of fruit sugars, which is why it is considered a treat in my house. Some 100 percent juices have more sugar per ounce than Coca-Cola. For example, Welch's concord grape juice has 36 grams of sugar in 8 ounces. Coke? It has 26 grams in 8 ounces.

You want to cut calories in juice? Add some water. I will buy a carton of 100 percent orange juice, and either serve 4 ounces or less or pour half of it into a pitcher and fill it with water. You will be surprised how good this tastes after you get used to it—plus you'll save money.

Frozen Meals, Frozen Pizza, and Canned Soups

When you trust Con-Agra, Nestlé, or Campbell's to make you a meal, you have to be aware that they want you to buy their products again and again. What is the best way to make food taste delicious and potentially addictive? Add fat and salt, and people will love it.

I always check the grams of fat and sodium on these products before I look at anything else. When you do this with your favorites, you will be blown away by what is in one slice of your favorite frozen pizza or canned soup. Many of the recipes in this book, like macaroni and cheese (page 176) and cream of mushroom soup (page 172), are designed to replace these packaged favorites. Healthy can also be delicious, though it may take some getting used to if you have been eating frozen meals with 800 milligrams of salt and 20 grams of fat per serving.

When I do buy prepared soups and frozen meals, I aim for less than 400 milligrams of salt and 10 grams of fat per serving. They're not easy to find; I've gotten some Amy's and Kashi meals that fit the bill. The good news is now you have the information to make educated decisions about what you buy and feed your family.

PART 2

Recipes

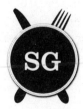

Philosophy

I want to inspire you to cook. Not by using fancy ingredients and time-consuming steps, but by creating recipes simple enough to make every day and tasty enough that you'll want to. I am attempting to make your life easier by providing the answer to the age-old question, "How do I get five to seven servings of fruits and vegetables every day?" My recipes almost always use a fruit or vegetable to make them less calorie dense and fill them with nutrients.

At the same time, I wanted to create recipes for foods that are comforting and recognizable, such as macaroni and cheese or chicken potpie.

When you use more vegetables, you can use less meat. By doing this you:

1. **Reduce calories and saturated fat.**

2. **Save money** (meat is more expensive per pound than vegetables).

3. **Go green.** Meat uses more resources than vegetables to reach the table, so when you eat less of it you are being environmentally friendly.

The type of dairy I use may surprise many who are used to diet recipes. I use whole milk, butter, whole-milk yogurt, sour cream, and Cheddar cheese almost exclusively. I do use less of it than in conventional recipes and I find that these whole-milk options taste better than their low-fat or nonfat counterparts. Healthy food has to taste good for you to want to make it over and over again.

I have done my best to keep the sodium in these recipes under control. If you are used to processed food, you may find these lower-sodium recipes lack flavor. Simply add more salt to taste. As you get used to home-cooked meals, you will need less salt for flavoring, but it takes time to adjust.

I do use frozen vegetables and some other processed foods. While I am sure we would all love to have the time to make homemade piecrust or tomato sauce, I know that isn't realistic for most of us on a daily basis. Do I want to rely on processed foods? No, but I do use some when things are hectic.

Many cookbooks are written without appreciating how difficult it is to clean up after making a meal. Not this one. Reducing cleanup time is very important to me because I hate scrubbing pans and washing dishes. Many of these meals can be made in one pan, pot, or bowl to minimize the post-cooking mess.

Finally, these recipes are as simple as I can make them. I have tested them to reduce them to as few steps possible. Please follow all of the steps. For example, if the recipe states "use parchment paper," it means I tried putting the food directly on the cookie sheet and it stuck so hard I had to use an ice pick to get it off. Therefore, get thee some parchment paper!

Recipes by Calories per Serving

This list is for the calorie counters who are experiencing success by monitoring their caloric intake.

UNDER 100 CALORIES

100 TO 200 CALORIES

Birthday Carrot Cake (page 262)

Apple Cake (page 266)

Upside-Down Sundae (page 269)

Cinnamon, Vanilla, and Sugar Roasted Almonds (page 270)

Hot, Thick, and Dark Chocolate Drink (page 272)

200 TO 300 CALORIES

Bacon, Egg, Cheese, and Onion Breakfast Burrito (page 136)

Beef, Black Bean, and Mushroom Burgers (page 146)

Slow Cooker Beef Stew (page 161)

Cocoa Chili (page 166)

White Chili (page 168)

Mexican Chicken Soup (page 169)

Sneaky Zucchini Lasagna (page 182)

Mighty Meatloaf (page 186)

Roasted Vegetables with Pasta (page 204)

Instant Banana Pudding (page 268)

300 TO 400 CALORIES

Hunter Slow Cooker Chicken Stew (page 160)

Slow Cooker Split Pea Soup (page 162)

Lentil Coconut Curry Stew (page 164)

Simplest Comforting Pasta (page 175)

Airy and Easy Mac and Cheese (page 176)

Beef and Veggie Cottage Pie (page 178)

Stovetop Tuna Casserole (page 181)

Chicken and Vegetable Potpie (page 184)

Roasted Vegetable Quesadilla (page 205)

Pantry List

Many Snack Girl readers find that they already have most of the ingredients for my recipes. The following list makes it easy to shop once a week and have everything you need to make simple meals.

When I mention a specific brand in this section, it is because I have had success using it. Also, it can be easier to find something when you have a brand to look for on the supermarket shelf. This list is not absolute; if you find another brand you like better, please use it (and send me an e-mail via Snack-Girl.com so I can learn about it!).

You can copy this list to take with you or download and print out a PDF from this link: www.snack-girl.com/pantry.pdf.

PRODUCE

Apples

Avocados

Bananas

Bell peppers, red and green

Broccoli

Carrots

Cauliflower

Celery

Garlic

Kale

Lemons

Mushrooms, presliced and washed (white or whatever is in stock)

Onions, yellow

Potatoes, russet, red-skinned

Scallions

Sweet Potatoes

Zucchini

BREAD

100% whole-wheat bread
100% whole-wheat tortillas

MEAT AND EGGS

Chicken breast, boneless, skinless
Eggs, local
Ground beef, 80% lean, 85% lean, and 90% lean
Ham hocks, smoked

DAIRY AND DAIRY SUBSTITUTES

Almond milk, unsweetened
Butter, unsalted
Milk, whole
Parmesan cheese, block
Sharp Cheddar cheese, block
Sour cream
Yogurt, plain whole-milk

FREEZER

Asian stir-fry vegetables
Berries, mixed
Blueberries
Broccoli, chopped
Carrot slices
Cauliflower
Corn kernels
Fillo pastry shells, mini
Mango pieces

Peas

Spinach, whole-leaf

Vegetables, mixed (corn, carrots, green beans)

PANTRY

Almonds, whole, sliced, and blanched (see Note, page 119)

Almond butter

Applesauce, unsweetened

Baking powder

Baking soda

Beans, canned (black, pinto, white, garbanzo, and kidney)

Canola oil

Chicken stock, low-sodium

Cocoa powder, unsweetened, such as Hershey's Special Dark

Coconut, dried (sweetened and unsweetened)

Dates, pitted

Dijon mustard

Flour, all-purpose

Flour, white whole wheat, such as King Arthur

Honey

Maple syrup

Mayonnaise

Nonstick cooking spray

Oats, quick, unflavored, such as Quaker Oats

Oats, whole rolled

Olive oil, extra-virgin

Pasta, 100% whole wheat (elbow, penne, spaghetti)

Peanut butter, creamy and chunky, all natural (no sugar or oil added)

Popcorn

Pumpkin puree, canned

Raisins

Sugar (white, dark brown, light brown)

Tomatoes, canned (diced, whole, crushed, low sodium)

Tuna, canned, packed in water

SPICES

Chili powder

Cinnamon, ground

Cumin, ground

Curry powder

Paprika, smoked

Pepper, black, whole peppercorns and ground

Thyme, dried

Vanilla extract

Note: Most unsalted almonds in the supermarket are dry roasted. If I indicate raw (unroasted) almonds, please use them for the recipe. Look in the baking section for raw almonds.

Five Pantry Meals

All of the ingredients for these five meals can be stored in your refrigerator, cupboard, or freezer for two weeks or more. Keep the meat in your freezer and thaw it in your refrigerator or microwave when you want to use it.

1. Cocoa Chili (page 166)
2. White Chili (page 168)
3. Simplest Comforting Pasta (page 175)
4. Stovetop Tuna Casserole (page 181)
5. Broccoli, Potato, and Cheese Chowder (without scallions) (page 170)

The list below contains all the ingredients you need to make these dishes. Whenever you run out of one, make sure to pick it up the next time you go to the store. I have a sticky note pad on my fridge so I write it down before I forget we are out of it.

FIVE-MEAL SHOPPING LIST

1 pound 80% lean ground beef

1 pound boneless, skinless chicken breast

8 ounces sour cream

An 8-ounce block sharp Cheddar cheese

A 4-ounce block Parmesan cheese

1 (8-ounce) potato

1 lemon

2 pounds frozen chopped broccoli

1 pound frozen peas

1 pound frozen carrot slices

2 pounds frozen Asian stir-fry vegetables

3 (15-ounce) cans pinto, kidney, or black beans

4 (15-ounce) cans white beans

1 (28-ounce) can crushed or whole plum tomatoes

1 can low-sodium cream of mushroom soup (such as Campbell's)

16 ounces low-sodium chicken broth

1 pound 100% whole-wheat elbow macaroni

Unsweetened cocoa powder

Ground cumin

Chili powder

Canola oil

Breakfast

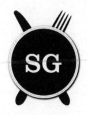

Boxed Pancake Mix Upgrade

**Makes 7 pancakes,
1 per serving**

**1 medium banana, mashed
(about ⅓ cup)**

**½ cup plain yogurt
(low fat or whole milk)**

1 large egg

**1 cup frozen blueberries,
thawed with juice**

**¾ cup 100% whole-wheat
pancake mix such as Hodgson
Mill Whole Wheat Buttermilk
Pancake Mix**

**Nonstick spray or butter,
as needed**

Hey, I know how busy things get and while we would all love to have the time to measure flour, sugar, and baking powder, life gets out of control. This recipe uses a 100 percent whole-wheat pancake mix as a shortcut.

I used Hodgson Mill Whole Wheat Buttermilk Pancake Mix because it was the only one on the shelf that was 100 percent whole wheat and the ingredient list was short. Whatever you buy, make sure it says *100 percent whole wheat*, not just *whole wheat*.

Banana, yogurt, and blueberries give the mix added flavor, fiber, and nutrition. I did not include any oil because you don't need it. You can always fry these in some butter to give them more flavor (and fat) if you want.

These make a great snack and keep well in the fridge for the next morning if you make too many. I like to use them for lunch with some peanut butter—peanut butter pancake sandwich, yum!

In a medium bowl, mash the banana with a fork until it is almost a liquid. Add the yogurt, egg, blueberries with juice, and pancake mix. Mix well.

Heat a nonstick griddle or frying pan over medium-high heat. Grease the pan with non-stick spray or a small pat of butter to keep the pancakes from sticking. Using a ladle, pour small circles of batter into the pan. Cook for a few minutes, until bubbles form on the top of the pancakes. Flip the pancakes and cook until firm.

Eat hot, warm, room temperature, or cold.

96 calories | 1.6 g fat | 0 g saturated fat | 18.1 g carbohydrates | 6.0 g sugar
5.3 g protein | 2.6 g fiber | 125 mg sodium

Overnight Pancakes

¾ cup whole-grain flour
(wheat, oat, etc.)

¾ cup rolled oats
(not instant)

1 teaspoon baking soda

½ teaspoon salt

1 tablespoon sugar

½ cup plain whole-milk yogurt

¾ cup whole milk

2 large eggs

Nonstick spray or butter,
as needed

If you need a hot breakfast that is fast and filling, these pancakes are a great solution.

The "overnight" part of this recipe is important because the oats get softer when they soak up the milk. They add a nice texture when you get around to making the pancakes.

You can leave this batter in the fridge for a couple of days and then cook as needed, or make it all at once and pop the leftover pancakes in the microwave to reheat. These are perfect for a before-school hot breakfast or a snack.

I calculated the nutrition facts using whole milk and whole-milk yogurt. The calories don't change very much with the low-fat or fat-free versions. Just use whatever you have on hand.

In a large bowl, stir the flour, oats, baking soda, salt, sugar, yogurt, milk, and eggs until well mixed. Cover the bowl and place in the refrigerator overnight.

In the morning, heat a nonstick griddle or frying pan over medium-high heat. Grease the pan with nonstick spray or a small pat of butter to keep the pancakes from sticking. Pour about ¼ cup batter for each pancake onto the pan and cook until bubbles begin showing on the surface. Flip and cook until firm.

---

104 calories | 2.6 g fat | 1.1 g saturated fat | 15.6 g carbohydrates | 1.0 g sugar
3.3 g protein | 1.0 g fiber | 296 mg sodium

Pumpkin Overnight Pancakes

**Makes 10 pancakes,
1 per serving**

¾ cup whole-grain flour (wheat,
oat, etc.)

¾ cup rolled oats (not instant)

1 teaspoon baking soda

1 teaspoon pumpkin pie spice

2 tablespoons sugar

1¾ cups whole milk

¾ cup canned pureed pumpkin

2 large eggs

Nonstick spray or butter,
as needed

Mix the flour, oats, baking soda, pumpkin pie spice, sugar, milk, pumpkin, and eggs together in a large bowl. Cover the bowl and refrigerate overnight.

In the morning, heat a nonstick griddle or frying pan over medium-high heat. Grease the pan with nonstick spray or a small pat of butter to keep the pancakes from sticking. Pour about ¼ cup batter for each pancake onto the pan and cook until bubbles begin showing on the surface. Flip and cook until firm.

---

116 calories | 3.1 g fat | 1.2 g saturated fat
18.0 g carbohydrates | 5.6 g sugar | 4.9 g protein
2.4 g fiber | 156 mg sodium

Easy Peasy Baked Oatmeal Muffins

**Makes 12 muffins,
1 per serving**

Nonstick spray

**2 cups rolled oats
(not instant)**

½ teaspoon baking powder

¼ teaspoon salt

1 teaspoon allspice

½ teaspoon ground cinnamon

2½ cups sliced fruit

1 cup whole milk

1 cup plain whole-milk yogurt

2 large eggs

**¼ cup maple syrup, honey, brown
sugar, or white sugar**

Make these ahead for a fast breakfast that elevates boring oatmeal. You can use any fruit that you have lying around your kitchen.

I like to use frozen blueberries, frozen mango pieces, or whole frozen blackberries because I don't want to do any slicing. I'm lazy like that. You don't have to thaw the fruit before you add it to the batter.

Preheat the oven to 350°F. Spray a 12-cup muffin tin with nonstick spray.

In a large bowl, mix the rolled oats, baking powder, salt, allspice, and cinnamon. Add the fruit, milk, yogurt, eggs, and maple syrup and stir until combined.

Divide the batter among the muffin cups and cover the muffin tin with foil. Bake for 20 minutes, remove the foil, and bake for another 25 minutes, or until golden brown and a toothpick inserted in the center of a muffin comes out clean.

Enjoy hot, cold, or at room temperature. If well covered, the muffins will keep in the fridge for one week.

---

128 calories | 3.2 g fat | 1.2 g saturated fat

19.7 g carbohydrates | 7.8 g sugar | 4.9 g protein

2.2 g fiber | 79 mg sodium

Reasonable Blueberry Muffins

**Makes 16 muffins,
1 per serving**

---

2 cups white whole-wheat flour,
such as King Arthur

⅓ cup sugar

½ teaspoon salt

1 tablespoon baking powder

1 teaspoon ground cinnamon

3 tablespoons canola oil

1 large egg, lightly beaten

1½ cups unsweetened
almond milk

1 cup frozen blueberries
(not thawed)

I think we have all met the unreasonable blueberry muffin. You find it at the convenience store or supermarket bakery. It is supersized, packed with calories, sugar, and fat, and has a large top that adds to our own muffin top.

This "reasonable" muffin sports no top at all (the shame!) and, with a smidge over 100 calories per muffin, is a much better way to start your day.

This recipe features King Arthur white whole-wheat flour, which you can find in the baking section of your grocery store. This flour is whole-wheat, which means it has all the nutrition from the wheat berry, but it is a lighter grain so your baked goods turn out fluffier without that overwhelming and sometimes bitter whole-wheat taste. My children don't even know that these are made with whole-wheat flour.

This recipe is lower in sugar and fat than a regular muffin recipe. I use unsweetened almond milk, which can be found in the dairy section of your supermarket. Almond milk has only 40 calories per cup and has a pleasingly nutty taste. If you don't have almond milk, use whatever milk you have in the house.

Preheat the oven to 400°F. Line a 12-cup muffin tin and 4 cups of another tin with paper liners. In the empty wells of the second tin, pour 1 tablespoon water to keep the tin from burning or warping.

In a large bowl, mix the flour, sugar, salt, baking powder, and cinnamon. Form a well in the center of the mixture.

In a medium bowl, mix together the oil, egg, and almond milk until combined. Pour the mixture into the well of the dry ingredients and add the frozen blueberries. Mix until just blended.

Fill the muffin cups two-thirds full. Bake for 20 to 25 minutes, until lightly browned and a toothpick inserted in the center of a muffin comes out clean.

BLUEBERRY LEMON MUFFINS

Add ½ teaspoon grated lemon zest to the oil, egg, and almond milk mixture. Yum!

---

103 calories | 3.5 g fat | 0.3 g saturated fat | 16.7 g carbohydrates
5.6 g sugar | 2.5 g protein | 1.9 g fiber | 94 mg sodium

Zucchini, Banana, and Almond Breakfast Muffins

**Makes 16 muffins,
1 per serving**

Nonstick spray

**1½ cups white whole-wheat flour
(such as King Arthur)**

⅓ cup packed light brown sugar

1 teaspoon baking soda

1 teaspoon baking powder

¼ teaspoon salt

1 teaspoon ground cinnamon

**1 small zucchini, coarsely grated
(about 1½ cups)**

**1 medium banana, mashed
(about ⅓ cup)**

½ cup chopped almonds

¾ cup whole milk

1 large egg

1 teaspoon vanilla extract

How do you make your muffins tender? How about a stick of butter? Yes, that is an easy way to get scrumptious muffins, but you can also get the same results with fruits and vegetables.

Zucchini imparts a lovely texture without adding any "vegetable" flavor. The banana also adds moisture as well as some sweetness. Combined, you get incredibly moist muffins.

Make these ahead so you can grab and go when you are off to work or school. I toss one in my lunchbox for my coffee break so I don't buy a large cookie.

Be sure to coat the cups of the muffin tins with the nonstick spray. When I baked these in paper liners, they stuck and I had to suck the muffin off the liner. When these come out of the oven, use a knife around the outside of the cup to free them gently.

Feel free to substitute whatever nuts you like instead of almonds to pack more nutrition into these muffins.

Preheat the oven to 375°F. Spray 16 muffin cups with nonstick spray. In the empty wells of the tin, pour 1 tablespoon water to keep the tin from burning or warping.

In a large bowl, mix the flour, sugar, baking soda, baking powder, salt, and cinnamon. Add the zucchini, banana, almonds, milk, egg, and vanilla, and stir until combined.

Divide the batter among the muffin cups and bake for 20 to 25 minutes, until a toothpick inserted in the center of a muffin comes out clean.

These store well in the freezer if you individually wrap them in plastic.

---

90 calories | 2.4 g fat | 0.4 g saturated fat | 15.3 g carbohydrates | 6.2 g sugar
3.1 g protein | 1.8 g fiber | 124 mg sodium

Do-It-Yourself Cereal Bars

**Makes 12 bars,
1 per serving**

Nonstick spray

**½ cup whole nuts
(choose your favorite)**

**1½ cups dried fruits
(cherries, cranberries, apricots,
raisins, coconut, etc.)**

**½ cup peanut butter or other
nut butter**

**2 medium bananas, mashed
(about ⅔ cup)**

**1 cup rolled oats
(not instant)**

**1 teaspoon vanilla extract
(optional)**

**Pinch of cinnamon
(optional)**

**¼ cup pumpkin
or sunflower seeds
(optional)**

This is one of the most popular recipes on the Snack Girl site—it's easy to make and solves a big breakfast dilemma. (Okay, they're not literally bars; I bake them in a muffin tin so they're easy to grab/store/freeze.) Many of us buy packaged cereal bars because we don't have time to make breakfast, but we feel bad because we know they have a lot of added sugar.

Never buy packaged cereal bars again!!

These get their sweetness from dried fruit and bananas instead of sugar. They *are* sweet—and also filling because of the peanut butter and nuts. Use any type of nut butter, such as almond butter, if you are allergic to peanuts. Also, any type of nuts or dried fruit will be delicious.

I calculated the nutrition facts using ½ cup almonds and 1½ cups raisins. Raisins have 16.8 grams of sugar per ounce, which is very high for dried fruit. I chose all raisins to err on the side of the most sugar and calories these bars could have. Try mixing in some lower-sugar dried fruits with the raisins (or dropping them entirely) to create these bars. For example, when I use dried apricots, the sugar is reduced from 13.7 grams to 4.8 grams per serving.

Individually wrap and freeze the bars to keep them fresh.

Preheat the oven to 350°F. Spray a 12-cup muffin tin with nonstick spray.

In a food processor, coarsely chop the nuts and dried fruits or chop by hand. In a large bowl, mix the peanut butter and bananas until a paste forms. Add the fruit and nuts, rolled oats, and any optional ingredients you desire and mix. Spoon into the muffin cups and bake for 15 minutes. Wrapped well, these can be stored in the refrigerator for 5 days or frozen for one month.

WITHOUT PUMPKIN OR SUNFLOWER SEEDS

187 calories | 7.9 g fat | 1.1 g saturated fat | 26.3 g carbohydrates | 13.7 g sugar

4.8 g protein | 3.0 g fiber | 38 mg sodium

Green Eggs

Serves 2,
1 cup per serving

---

1 cup frozen whole-leaf spinach

3 large eggs

1 ounce sharp Cheddar cheese, grated

If you love Dr. Seuss's *Green Eggs and Ham*, you are going to get a kick out of these eggs. They are (dare I say it?) fun.

My mother thought this concept was a bit strange but I got her to try them. Just close your eyes and you will be convinced.

By adding a cup of frozen spinach to these eggs, you add an additional 3.8 grams of protein and 10 percent of your daily value of iron per serving. The extra nutrients from the spinach make this a "super breakfast." You will grab a cape after eating it (or maybe you will just smile as you start your car).

Serve the eggs with toast or wrap them in a whole-wheat tortilla.

Using a blender, puree the spinach, 2 tablespoons water, and the eggs. The mixture will seem watery for an omelet or scrambled eggs, but don't be concerned; it will come together as it cooks.

Heat a nonstick frying pan over medium-high heat and pour the mixture into the hot pan. Sprinkle the cheese over the eggs and either flip for an omelet or stir to scramble them.

Serve immediately. These will store, covered, in the fridge for a few days but only taste good when hot.

187 calories | 12.3 g fat | 5.5 g saturated fat | 5.6 g carbohydrates | 1.0 g sugar
15.4 g protein | 3.5 g fiber | 283 mg sodium

Bacon, Egg, Cheese, and Onion Breakfast Burrito

Serves 6,
½ burrito per serving

---

6 slices center-cut bacon

1 large onion, sliced

6 large eggs

3 ounces sharp Cheddar cheese, grated

3 large whole-wheat tortillas

This recipe was inspired by a McDonald's bacon, Cheddar, and onion burger. I thought, "Hey, that sounds delicious!"

These are super easy to make, but they take some organization. I use one pan and cook the bacon, onion, and egg one after the other, then mix them together to fill the tortillas. Add other vegetables to the mix if you like them. Mushrooms work well here as does any roasted vegetable (page 191) you have in your fridge.

Center-cut bacon has less fat per serving than regular bacon and all of the flavor. I am not a fan of turkey bacon, but it is an okay substitute if you prefer it.

These have just over 200 calories per serving. Pair one with an apple as you walk out the door.

Lay the bacon slices in a large frying pan. Cook over medium heat until crispy. Drain the bacon on paper towels and then chop into small pieces. Pour the bacon fat out of the pan.

Add the onion to the hot pan and cook, stirring frequently, until browned, about 10 minutes. Put the cooked onion in a small bowl and set aside. In a large bowl, whisk the eggs with 2 tablespoons water until frothy. Scramble the eggs in the same hot pan.

In a large bowl, mix the scrambled eggs, bacon, onion, and cheese. Place one third of the filling (about ¾ cup) along the center of each tortilla.

Fold in the short ends, then fold the long ends over the filling. Lay the burrito folded side down and, using a very sharp serrated knife, cut it in half. If not eating right away, wrap the halves in plastic and store in the fridge or freezer for a grab-and-go breakfast. To reheat, put on a plate and microwave on high for 30 to 60 seconds if not frozen, or for 1½ minutes if frozen.

---

208 calories | 11.1 g fat | 4.9 g saturated fat | 13.9 g carbohydrates | 1.5 g sugar
13.7 g protein | 1.9 g fiber | 306 mg sodium

Baked Eggs and Cheese in Toast Cups

Serves 1

**¼ teaspoon butter
(salted or unsalted)**

**1 slice 100%
whole-wheat bread**

**1 tablespoon grated sharp
Cheddar cheese**

1 medium egg

Salt and pepper to taste

If you grab your breakfast on the road, then this recipe will help you stop that habit. Call me a traditionalist, but I like to have eggs and toast in the morning.

These are *so* much fun to make. All you do is shove bread into a buttered muffin tin or ramekin, then drop in some cheese and a medium egg. My kids get a kick out of making these; anyone over the age of eight can make them. I precook six of them on the weekend for the crazy week ahead.

These are best made in ramekins, which are small glazed ceramic dishes. If you don't own any, you can always find them at thrift stores because, for some reason, people don't use them and they give them away.

When I want breakfast, I just put some plastic wrap over the finished product—still in the ramekin—then heat it in the microwave for a minute or two and enjoy!

Preheat the oven to 375°F. Soften the butter in the microwave (if using a ramekin, just put it in the dish). Using a paper towel, butter the dish so the toast will not stick.

Squeeze the bread into the cup, tearing it a bit to make it fit. Push the bread against the sides of the cup to make space for the cheese and egg.

Sprinkle the grated cheese into the bread cup and add the egg. For a runny egg, bake for 15 minutes; for a half-soft, half-hard yolk, bake for 20 minutes; and for fully cooked, bake for 25 minutes.

Add salt and pepper and serve.

If you make a bunch of these ahead of time, store them wrapped in plastic wrap in your refrigerator for one week.

---

165 calories | 8.7 g fat | 3.7 g saturated fat | 12.9 g carbohydrates | 2.4 g sugar

10.3 g protein | 3.0 g fiber | 262 mg sodium

Mains

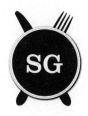

Burgers, Salads, and Tacos

Sweet Potato, Bean, and Corn Burger

We all get bored with the same old turkey sandwich for lunch. This very low fat "burger" is vegan, yummy, and great with lettuce and tomato slices. You could also put guacamole on top or serve it on a bed of rice.

I bake the sweet potatoes the night before I'm going to make the burgers and refrigerate them, wrapped in aluminum foil. You can also cook the potatoes in a microwave.

After you cook the burgers, put a few on a baking sheet and set them in the freezer. When they're frozen, wrap them individually in plastic wrap and store them for up to one month. They will be a little soggy after being frozen and reheated in a microwave or toaster oven, but you can add back some crunch with lettuce.

If you don't have instant oats, pulse your whole oats in a food processor a couple of times to get the right consistency for this recipe.

**Makes 12 burgers,
1 (5-ounce) burger per serving**

**2 pounds sweet potatoes
(about 3 large potatoes)**

Nonstick spray

**1 (15-ounce) can black beans
(preferably low sodium)**

**½ cup corn kernels,
fresh or frozen (thawed)**

1 small onion, diced

1 large garlic clove, minced

1 cup instant oats

1 tablespoon chili powder

1 teaspoon salt

BAKE THE SWEET POTATOES

Oven method: Preheat the oven to 350°F and prick the sweet potatoes a couple of times with a fork. Place them on a baking sheet lined with aluminum foil. Bake for 1 hour, or until very soft. At this point you can store the sweet potatoes for a couple of days until you are ready to make the burgers.

Microwave method: Prick the sweet potatoes a couple of times with a fork, wrap in a paper towel, and place on a microwave-safe plate. Cook on high for 5 minutes, turn over, and cook for another 5 minutes, until soft.

MAKE THE BURGERS

Preheat the oven to 375°F and spray a baking sheet with nonstick spray. Drain the black beans, put half of them in a large bowl, and mash with a potato masher. Peel the sweet potatoes with your hands. The skins should come right off if they have been baked long enough.

Add the potatoes to the bowl with the mashed black beans and mash them together. Add the whole black beans, corn, onion, garlic, oats, chili powder, and salt. Mix until combined and then make twelve burger patties with your hands ½ to ¾ inch thick. Place the patties on the baking sheet.

Bake for 15 minutes and flip the burgers. Bake for another 15 minutes and enjoy!

---

143 calories | 1.0 g fat | 0 g saturated fat | 29.2 g carbohydrates | 4.2 g sugar | 5.5 g protein
6.6 g fiber | 248 mg sodium

Beef, Black Bean, and Mushroom Burgers

**Makes 9 burgers,
1 (6-ounce) burger per serving**

**1 (15-ounce) can black beans,
drained and rinsed**

**1 (8-ounce) package
presliced and washed
white mushrooms**

**1⅓ pounds 85% lean
ground beef**

3 large eggs

½ teaspoon salt

This compromise between a veggie burger and a hamburger is meaty, satisfying, and pretty healthy. A 6-ounce hamburger made with 85% lean ground beef has 435 calories. My creative beef, black bean, and mushroom burger has 247 calories, good stuff like fiber, and less than half the saturated fat. One key to success is to mash up the beans until they are not recognizable. I got lazy one day and my daughter asked me about the raisin in her burger. "No, honey, that's not a raisin, it's a bean," I said. She decided right then she wasn't going to eat it.

Hopefully, you will have more luck with your family.

In a large bowl, mash the black beans with a potato masher until mostly crushed. Chop the mushrooms into small chunks. Mix the beef, mushrooms, eggs, and salt into the mashed beans with your hands until blended. Shape the mixture into 9 patties.

Heat a nonstick pan over medium-high heat. Cook the burgers for 3 minutes, flip, and cook for another 3 minutes. Flip again and after a couple more minutes, check to see if the burgers are pink. After about 10 minutes, the burgers will be cooked through.

Serve on a bun with tomato, lettuce, cheese, mayonnaise, ketchup, or mustard, if desired.

WITHOUT THE BUN OR TOPPINGS

247 calories | 12.2 g fat | 4.4 g saturated fat | 8.9 g carbohydrates | 0.5 g sugar
24.4 g protein | 2.9 g fiber | 216 mg sodium

Tastiest Turkey Burgers

**Makes 6 burgers,
1 (3-ounce) burger per serving**

1 large bunch fresh cilantro,
stemmed (1 to 1½ cups loosely
packed leaves)

1 pound 93% lean ground turkey

1 bunch scallions (5 to 6), both
white and green parts, chopped

1 tablespoon curry powder

½ teaspoon salt

Lean ground turkey is considered a healthier source of protein for a burger than ground beef because it has fewer calories per ounce. You have to be sure to buy the 93% lean turkey because regular ground turkey has as much saturated fat and calories as lean ground beef.

I must admit to hating turkey burgers for most of my adult life because I found them bland. But these burgers are delicious and you won't even notice that they aren't beef. I use a mixture of scallions, cilantro, and curry powder to make these burgers sing with flavor.

I hate buying fresh herbs or scallions and then watching them turn to slimy sludge in my fridge. When a recipe calls for 1 tablespoon of chopped sage, I always wonder what I am going to do with the rest of it.

This recipe uses all of the scallions and cilantro in the bunches that you buy from the store. Don't worry if the measurement isn't exact—just use it all up and feel good about the mess that didn't result in your vegetable drawer.

Wash and chop all of the leaves from the bunch of cilantro. In a large bowl, mix the cilantro, turkey, scallions, curry powder, and salt. Make 6 burger patties and place on a plate.

Heat a nonstick pan over medium heat. When hot, add the burgers; cook 2 minutes and flip. Keep flipping every 2 minutes until the burgers are no longer pink in the center. They will cook through in about 8 minutes.

Serve on a bun with tomatoes, lettuce, mayonnaise, and/or ketchup, if desired. Or put them in a pita with a squirt of lime and avocado slices.

WITHOUT THE BUN OR TOPPINGS

111 calories | 5.5 g fat | 1.7 g saturated fat | 0.7 g carbohydrates | 0 g sugar

14.9 g protein | 0 g fiber | 252 mg sodium

Lightest Tuna Melt

Serves 4,
½ pepper per serving

---

1 (5-ounce) can tuna packed in water, drained

1 tablespoon mayonnaise

2 celery stalks, chopped

2 scallions, both white and green parts, sliced

Salt and pepper to taste

2 medium red bell peppers, halved, core and seeds removed

2 ounces Cheddar cheese, cut into 4 small slices

You know how everyone is always badmouthing carbohydrates? I'm not one of those people.

However, I am a fan of eating as many fruits and vegetables as I can in one day. This tuna melt uses red peppers as a substitute for bread, and it works. Not only is it lovely to look at, you also get a soft, cheesy tuna flavor combined with a crunch of pepper.

I have decided that this version of a tuna melt is actually better without the bread.

If you don't have a red pepper or you find them to be too expensive, just use a slice of 100 percent whole-wheat bread as the base. You are still getting some vegetable goodness with the celery and scallions mixed in.

Heat the broiler to high. Mix the tuna, mayonnaise, celery, and scallions in a small bowl. Season with a little salt and pepper. Divide the mixture among the pepper halves and top each with a slice of cheese. Place the peppers on a rimmed baking sheet and roast under the broiler for 3 minutes or until the cheese is melted.

The cooked peppers can be stored in the refrigerator for up to 3 days.

135 calories | 6.4 g fat | 3.3 g saturated fat | 5.4 g carbohydrates | 3.1 g sugar
13.4 g protein | 1.6 g fiber | 264 mg sodium

Ham and Cheese Zucchiniwich

Serves 1

---

1 medium zucchini

1 ounce sharp Cheddar cheese

1 slice ham (about 1 ounce)

½ teaspoon Dijon mustard (optional)

This "zucchiniwich" has 57 percent of your daily value of vitamin C, 24 percent of your daily value of calcium, and 7 percent of your daily value of iron.

The zucchini lends just 31 calories to the sandwich versus bread, which is usually around 100 calories per slice or 200 for the sandwich. Make a few of these and store them in a plastic container to take to work. They reheat well in a microwave (after you have broiled them at home) and will not leave you with that heavy feeling after lunch.

The sodium here is high because I use ham. If you can find low-sodium ham or other low-sodium cold cuts (such as turkey or chicken breast), use them for a less salty version.

You can pick these up just like a regular sandwich and shove them in your mouth. Yum!

Slice the zucchini lengthwise and remove the seeds by running a small spoon down the center to create a shallow "canoe" for the filling. Place on a plate and microwave for 2 minutes on high to soften. While the zucchini is cooking, chop the cheese and ham into small pieces and mix together in a bowl with the Dijon (if using). Stuff the hollowed-out zucchini halves with the mixture.

Heat a broiler or toaster oven to high and cook for 2 minutes, or until the cheese is melted. Let cool for a minute before eating so you don't burn your mouth.

---

192 calories | 12.2 g fat | 6.9 g saturated fat | 8.0 g carbohydrates | 3.5 g sugar

14.1 g protein | 2.5 g fiber | 565 mg sodium

Healthy Tacos with a Twist

Makes 12 tacos,
1 per serving

8 ounces 90% lean ground beef

1 (8-ounce) package presliced and washed white mushrooms, chopped

1 cup frozen (unthawed) or fresh (uncooked) corn kernels

1 package taco seasoning mix

12 hard taco shells

Optional toppings

Fresh salsa

Sliced avocado

Shredded lettuce

Grated Cheddar cheese

Chopped fresh tomatoes

1 (15-ounce) can black beans, rinsed and drained

My mother cannot cook but she can make tacos. They were a big treat growing up, and I still love them. They are usually made with a pound of ground beef, but I think tacos are a great VDD (Vegetable Delivery Device).

What child (or adult for that matter) is going to notice some mushrooms and corn mixed in with her ground meat? Even if they skip the tomato, avocado, and lettuce you provided and just load up on the cheese, they still get some veggies.

If you want to make this meal *super* healthy, don't eat the hard taco shells (they're really just large chips). Depending on the size of your taco shell, you can save 50 to 70 calories per taco by substituting lettuce. Choose romaine over iceberg if it's available. Romaine has much more beta-carotene, folate, and vitamin K, among other nutrients, than iceberg. Wash some lettuce, shred it, and add all your toppings to make a taco salad that will convince you never to visit Taco Bell again.

I used taco seasoning mix as an ingredient because it's easy to find and use, but it is high in sodium. Buy a low-sodium mix or make your own: Combine 2 teaspoons cumin, 1 tablespoon chili powder, a minced garlic clove, and ½ teaspoon salt (or no salt) and you will have something that tastes much the same. Do not add any water if you make your own mix.

It can be difficult to buy just 8 ounces (½ pound) of ground beef as most super-market packages contain at least a pound. You can ask the store butcher to make you an 8-ounce package or you can just double the recipe and freeze the filling that you don't eat. That way you have a meal ready to go for those busy nights.

Heat a nonstick skillet to high. Add the beef and cook, stirring to break up the meat, until browned. Drain off the fat. Add the mushrooms, corn, taco seasoning mix, and ⅔ cup water. Heat to boiling, reduce the heat, and simmer uncovered for 3 to 4 minutes. Warm up the taco shells using package directions. Load the taco shells with the filling and add optional fixings.

WITHOUT TOPPINGS

116 calories | 4.7 g fat | 1.4 g saturated fat | 11.8 g carbohydrates | 0.7 g sugar

6.5 g protein | 0.8 g fiber | 344 mg sodium

WITH TOPPINGS

(1 tablespoon grated Cheddar cheese, 1 tablespoon fresh salsa, ¼ cup shredded lettuce,

1 small slice avocado, ¼ cup chopped tomato, and 1 tablespoon black beans)

213 calories | 8.6 g fat | 3.1 g saturated fat | 23.1 g carbohydrates | 2.8 g sugar

11.8 g protein | 4.2 g fiber | 488 mg sodium

Poached Boneless, Skinless Chicken Breast for Every Day

**Serves 4,
4 ounces per serving**

---

1 pound boneless, skinless chicken breasts (about 2)

2 teaspoons dried thyme

1 garlic clove

Skinless chicken breasts have the registered dietician seal of approval. They love the lean source of protein and its ease of use. Skinless chicken breast costs you a mere 1 gram of saturated fat for 26 grams of protein in one serving and is packed with nutrients. Wouldn't it be great if it tasted like filet mignon?

Alas, skinless chicken breast is boring and tasteless. On the other hand, it is easy to cook and very versatile if you can figure out how to flavor it. There are tons of recipes that include "cooked chicken meat" as an ingredient so it is helpful to have some ready to go.

You can use the poached chicken in a taco, chop it up and put it on a salad, or slice it for a sandwich. I use it in Chicken and Vegetable Potpie (page 184) and Simplest Chicken Salad (page 158).

This recipe is foolproof and one that you will use many times. Feel free to cook as many pounds as you want at once and then store in the fridge or freezer for later use.

Place the chicken in the bottom of a heavy pot. Cover with water by about ½ inch. Add the thyme and garlic.

Bring to a boil, then reduce the heat to a simmer. Partly cover the pot and simmer for 10 minutes. Remove the pot from the heat, cover, and let the chicken poach for 15 minutes.

Take the chicken out of the pot with tongs and slice on a cutting board to check for doneness. If it is too pink for your taste, put it back in the hot water until cooked through (another 5 minutes or so). Refrigerate the chicken whole or in chunks.

---

129 calories | 2.5 g fat | 0.5 g saturated fat | 0 g carbohydrates | 0 g sugar | 23 g protein
0 g fiber | 180 mg sodium

Simplest Chicken Salad

Chicken salad usually is just chicken with a little bit of vegetable and a whole lot of mayonnaise. In this recipe, I increased the vegetables and decreased the mayonnaise. I use real mayo, because the flavor is so much better than any low-fat variety, as well as Dijon mustard to add more creaminess with fewer calories.

Give this a try on a bed of lettuce, in a pita, or on whole-wheat sandwich bread. I keep a container of this in my fridge for an easy lunch; it will keep for a week.

Serves 6, ½ cup per serving

1 pound cooked chicken breast (see preceding recipe)

1 cup chopped celery (2 stalks)

1 cup chopped carrots (2 medium carrots)

¼ cup plus 1 tablespoon mayonnaise

2 tablespoons Dijon mustard

½ teaspoon dried thyme, basil, or oregano

¼ teaspoon salt, or more to taste

Black pepper

Chop the chicken breast into small pieces. Mix the chicken, celery, carrots, mayonnaise, mustard, thyme, and salt in a large bowl. Season with pepper to taste.

187 calories | 7.1 g fat | 1.4 g saturated fat
5.6 g carbohydrates | 2.1 g sugar | 24.1 g protein | 1.1 g fiber
328 mg sodium

Stew, Chili, and Soup

Hunter Slow Cooker Chicken Stew

Do you find yourself hunting for a way to make dinner without a lot of work? Well, this take on a *cacciatore*, or hunter's stew, is the perfect solution to your problem.

The slow cooker does all of the work here, fusing the flavors of the chicken, mushrooms, pepper, onion, and tomatoes to create a dish of wonderful depth.

You can serve this over pasta or rice or just with a slice of bread on the side.

Serves 5, 2 cups per serving

1½ pounds boneless, skinless chicken thighs

1 (8-ounce) package presliced and washed white mushrooms

1 green pepper, sliced

1 medium onion, sliced

3 large carrots, peeled and cut into ½-inch chunks

2 garlic cloves, peeled and minced

1 (28-ounce) can crushed tomatoes

1 teaspoon dried oregano

Salt and pepper to taste

Place the chicken, mushrooms, green pepper, onion, carrots, garlic, tomatoes, and oregano in a 6-quart slow cooker. Cover and cook on the low setting for 7 hours. Taste just before serving and season with salt and pepper.

333 calories | 13.6 g fat | 3.7 g saturated fat

13.0 g carbohydrates | 6.7 g sugar | 37.7 g protein

3.9 g fiber | 292 mg sodium

Slow Cooker Beef Stew

**Serves 8,
1 ½ cups per serving**

---

1 ½ pounds beef round stew meat, cut into 1 ½-inch chunks

2 tablespoons balsamic vinegar

2 tablespoons all-purpose flour

1 (14.5-ounce) can diced tomatoes with no added salt

1 pound (4 medium) red-skinned potatoes, scrubbed and cut into 1 ½-inch chunks

½ pound (2 medium) onions, halved and cut into 1-inch pieces

1 pound carrots, peeled and sliced into 1-inch chunks

3 garlic cloves, peeled and smashed

2 bay leaves (optional)

Salt and pepper to taste

Stew is one of those comfort foods that can be good for you if you do it right. The key is to use more vegetables than beef.

This is a meal that I eat all winter long when I am craving cheese and red wine. With over 100 percent of my daily value of vitamin A and 18 percent of my iron, it is a lot better for me than Cabernet and Camembert.

You can usually find beef round cut into chunks for stew in the meat section of your supermarket. Add some frozen peas at the end and heat for five minutes in the stew to give a splash of green and even more vegetables!

Place the beef in a 6-quart slow cooker. Mix in the vinegar and flour. Pour the diced tomatoes with their juice on top of the beef.

Add the potatoes, onions, carrots, garlic, and bay leaves (if using) to the slow cooker, leaving the beef completely submerged at the bottom of the pot. Cook on low for 7 hours.

Remove the bay leaves, taste, and season with salt and pepper.

---

279 calories | 8.5 g fat | 3.1 g saturated fat

21.6 g carbohydrates | 6.2 g sugar | 28.3 g protein

4.0 g fiber | 117 mg sodium

Slow Cooker Split Pea Soup

**Serves 8,
1 ½ cups per serving**

---

1 pound green split peas

1 large onion, diced

2 large carrots, diced

**1 smoked ham hock (10 to 14
ounces)**

**3 garlic cloves, peeled and
smashed**

1 bay leaf (optional)

**½ teaspoon dried thyme
(optional)**

Salt and pepper to taste

This is classic comfort food with benefits. The benefits are a ton of protein, fiber, and vitamins. The comforts are the thick and creamy texture and meaty ham flavor. You can find ham hocks next to the ham in the meat section. They usually come in packages of three; I freeze the extra ones for later use.

Not only is this meal nutritious, it is also cheap. This is a standard in my house. When I add croutons, my children love this green soup. Without croutons, they complain.

You can buy croutons or make them yourself. Check out Snack-Girl.com for a simple crouton recipe.

Pour the peas into a strainer and rinse thoroughly. Check for small pebbles, then pour into a 6-quart slow cooker. Add the onion, carrots, ham hock, garlic, bay leaf and thyme (if using), and 2 quarts water and cook on low for 7 to 8 hours, until the peas are soft.

When the peas are soft, remove the ham hock and bay leaf. Puree the soup with a hand-held blender or pour into a regular blender to puree. This will take a few batches. Be sure not to overfill your blender or you will have a big mess on your hands.

Cut off any ham that remains on the hock, chop it into chunks, and put it back in the soup. Throw away the bone and fat that remain.

Depending on the saltiness of your ham hock, you may need to add 1 teaspoon or more of salt to make your soup taste delicious. The nutrition facts below reflect very little salt added, so do not fear adding salt. Lots of pepper makes this extra tasty.

Serve plain or with a few croutons.

WITHOUT CROUTONS

317 calories | 6.8 g fat | 2.3 g saturated fat | 38.1 g carbohydrates | 6.2 g sugar

26.7 g protein | 15.3 g fiber | 60 mg sodium

Lentil Coconut Curry Stew

**Serves 8,
1 ¼ cups per serving**

2 tablespoons vegetable oil

3 garlic cloves, minced

1-inch piece fresh ginger, peeled
and minced

2 medium onions, chopped

2 cups dried red lentils

3 medium carrots, chopped

1 (15-ounce) can coconut milk

1 teaspoon curry powder

1 teaspoon ground cumin

1 teaspoon salt

1 bay leaf (optional)

Can you make a hearty stew without meat? Absolutely. This one uses lentils and coconut milk to give it heft.

Red lentils, which you can find in the dried beans section of your grocery store (often next to the canned beans), can be cooked in 15 minutes. You don't need to presoak them and they are an excellent source of fiber and protein.

Coconut milk is very tasty. It does have saturated fat, but this type of saturated fat has health benefits as opposed to the fat in red meat. Do not fear it.

I use fresh ginger, which can be found in the produce section, because it gives such a nice flavor to the dish. If you can't find it, use ground ginger. Add a teaspoon of ground ginger while cooking and then more when the dish is finished to adjust the flavors to your liking.

Each serving has 27 percent of your daily value of iron, 9.5 grams of fiber, and 77 percent of your daily value of vitamin A.

The serving size is small here because the stew is thick. Change its consistency by blending it and adding vegetable broth and you have soup. Serve it with brown rice (page 212), cauliflower rice (page 214), or whole-wheat pasta.

Heat the oil in a large saucepan. Sauté the garlic, ginger, and onions until the onions are translucent. Add the lentils, carrots, coconut milk, 1 quart water, curry powder, cumin, salt, and bay leaf (if using). Cover and bring to a boil. Reduce the heat to a simmer and cook, uncovered, for 15 minutes, or until the lentils are tender.

Serve chunky or remove the bay leaf and puree in a blender for a smoother consistency.

---

346 calories | 16.8 g fat | 12.0 g saturated fat | 37.2 g carbohydrates | 5.0 g sugar
14.3 g protein | 9.5 g fiber | 323 mg sodium

Cocoa Chili

**Serves 10,
1 ¼ cups per serving**

---

1 pound 80% lean ground beef

1 (28-ounce) can plum tomatoes

**3 (15-ounce) cans beans
(black, kidney, white, pinto—your
choice), drained and rinsed**

**2 tablespoons good-quality
chili powder**

**2 tablespoons unsweetened
cocoa powder**

1 tablespoon ground cumin

Salt to taste

Hot sauce (optional)

Everybody has his or her favorite chili recipe; this is mine. It's one of my family's favorite meals. I delivered this chili to a friend of mine after she had a stroke, and she asked me to write it down because her kids loved it.

For years, I had been throwing the ingredients into the pot from my pantry and hoping for the best. So, I forced myself to slow down and measure, and write it all down.

This recipe was what I came up with. Sometimes the chili powder isn't strong enough; I have been known to add up to ¼ cup to make it taste like super chili.

Play with the seasonings and make it yours.

Brown the ground beef in a large saucepan over medium-high heat. When the meat is browned, drain the fat from the pan. Add the tomatoes with their juices, breaking up whole tomatoes with a wooden spoon. Add the beans, chili powder, cocoa, and cumin. Heat to a simmer and taste for salt. Add hot sauce if desired at this point, or pass it around at the table. Cook for about 10 minutes at a low simmer. Serve plain or over rice or pasta.

This chili improves in the fridge overnight and freezes well.

---

281 calories | 9.6 g fat | 3.1 g saturated fat | 25.8 g carbohydrates | 2.1 g sugar
22.5 g protein | 8.7 g fiber | 298 mg sodium

White Chili

Serves 8,
1 ½ cups per serving

---

2 cups low-sodium chicken broth

1 pound boneless, skinless chicken breasts, cut into ½-inch chunks

4 (15-ounce) cans cannellini beans (white beans), drained and rinsed

3 tablespoons chili powder

1 teaspoon ground cumin

Grated Cheddar cheese (optional)

If you are bored with beef chili, you can always try white chili.

White chili uses chicken as a base instead of beef and is usually swimming with sour cream and cheese. Instead of sour cream, I have used mashed white beans to get a creamy texture. You can add a little grated cheese to the bowl if you miss the dairy.

In a large saucepan, heat the chicken broth. Add the chicken and simmer for 10 minutes, or until cooked through.

In a large bowl, mash 2 cans (4 cups) of the white beans until they are chunky but not paste.

Add the mashed beans, whole beans, chili powder, and cumin to the chicken and broth. Simmer until hot, about 10 minutes, ladle into bowls, and sprinkle with cheese if you prefer.

WITHOUT CHEESE

299 calories | 1.8 g fat | 0 g saturated fat

41.9 g carbohydrates | 2.2 g sugar | 28.4 g protein

16.9 g fiber | 338 mg sodium

Mexican Chicken Soup

This is my favorite soup for getting over a cold; the chili powder and cumin give it a south-of-the-border flavor and it is packed with vegetables. It is fast to make and the spiciness clears my nasal passages. The Mayo Clinic says that chicken soup helps relieve cold and flu symptoms. Why not give it a try?

**Serves 5,
2 cups per serving**

2 teaspoons extra-virgin olive oil

1 medium onion, chopped

4 garlic cloves, minced

1 medium green pepper, chopped

1 quart low-sodium chicken broth

1 (14-ounce) can diced tomatoes, drained

1 pound boneless, skinless chicken breasts, chopped

2 cups frozen corn kernels

2 teaspoons ground cumin

2 teaspoons chili powder

Salt to taste

Crushed tortilla chips, for garnish (optional)

Grated Cheddar cheese, for garnish (optional)

Heat the olive oil in a large pot over medium heat. Add the onion, garlic, and green pepper and sauté until soft, about 7 minutes.

Add the chicken broth, tomatoes, chicken, corn, cumin, and chili powder to the pot and bring to a boil. Adjust to a simmer and cook until the chicken is cooked through, 12 to 15 minutes. Taste for salt and adjust the seasonings.

Garnish with crushed tortilla chips or shredded cheese if you want to bulk it up.

WITHOUT GARNISHES

216 calories | 4.8 g fat | 0.8 g saturated fat

19.9 g carbohydrates | 5.1 g sugar | 23.2 g protein

3.4 g fiber | 220 mg sodium

Broccoli, Potato, and Cheese Chowder

**Serves 4,
about 1 ½ cups per serving**

1 large potato (8 ounces), cut into
½-inch cubes

1 pound fresh broccoli, cut into
small florets, or 1 pound frozen
chopped broccoli

3 cups low-sodium chicken stock

2 ounces sharp Cheddar cheese,
grated

2 scallions, white and green
parts, minced

Do you like chowder? I am a fan of chowder versus soup because chowder feels more like a meal. This chowder is incredibly easy to make and packs 11 percent of your daily value of iron, 19 percent of your daily value of vitamin A, and 17 percent of your daily value of calcium in every serving. Crazy!

You do have to cook the fresh broccoli and potato before you finish the soup, but this step is easy. If you use frozen broccoli, you don't have to cook it as it has already been blanched.

You will be surprised how a little cheese goes a long way here. You can add it to the entire pot or just toss some grated cheese into your bowl for a French-onion-soup effect.

If using fresh broccoli: Bring 2 quarts water to a boil in a large saucepan. Add the potato and boil for 5 minutes. Add the broccoli and boil for another 5 minutes, or until both potato and broccoli are tender. Drain the vegetables and empty the saucepan.

In the same saucepan, heat the chicken stock. Add the broccoli, potato, cheese, and scallions. Heat until hot and serve.

If using frozen broccoli: Bring 1 quart water to a boil in a large saucepan. Add the potato and boil for 5 minutes. Drain the potato and empty the saucepan.

In the same saucepan, heat the chicken stock until simmering. Add the frozen broccoli, potato, cheese, and scallions. Simmer for 2 minutes. Serve.

Note: If you would like the chowder to be thicker, blend for about 10 seconds with an immersion blender. Alternatively, you can puree 1 cup (or more) of the soup in a blender, then add it back to the pot.

---

174 calories | 5.2 g fat | 3.0 g saturated fat | 23.6 g carbohydrates | 2.9 g sugar
10.4 g protein | 5.2 g fiber | 178 mg sodium

Almost Cream of Mushroom Soup

Serves 4,
about 2 cups per serving

2 tablespoons butter

2 (8-ounce) packages presliced
and washed white mushrooms

1 onion, chopped

1 garlic clove, minced

¼ cup all-purpose flour

1 quart low-sodium chicken broth

1 cup whole milk

1 teaspoon dried thyme

¼ teaspoon salt, or to taste

Sadly, most canned cream of mushroom soup is very high in sodium and fat. So if you love it, give this recipe a try.

This soup is ridiculously fast to make if you buy presliced and cleaned fresh mushrooms. I used white mushrooms, but you can use whatever mushrooms you prefer.

This soup is a nutritional powerhouse. It is high in iron (24 percent of your daily value), niacin, phosphorus, and vitamin B_6. You won't even notice the health benefits because it tastes so much better than the canned version.

You need to keep stirring when you add the flour and then the liquid ingredients. If you don't stir enough, you will get little lumps of flour in your soup.

Melt the butter in a large frying pan. Sauté the mushrooms, onion, and garlic until the onion is translucent, about 7 minutes. Add the flour and stir until it turns light brown (about 2 minutes).

Add the chicken broth, stirring as you add it. Heat to a simmer, then stir in the milk, thyme, and salt to taste. Enjoy!

167 calories | 8.2 g fat | 4.8 g saturated fat | 16.4 g carbohydrates | 6.3 g sugar | 8 g protein
1.9 g fiber | 287 mg sodium

Pasta and Casseroles

Simplest Comforting Pasta

**Serves 4,
about 1 ½ cups per serving**

8 ounces 100% whole-wheat cut pasta, such as penne, elbows, or rigatoni

2 teaspoons vegetable oil (such as canola) or extra-virgin olive oil

2 pounds frozen Asian stir-fry vegetables

¼ cup sour cream

½ lemon

Chopped parsley or other fresh herbs (optional)

Salt and pepper to taste

This is one of those recipes that will stop you from ordering takeout when you drag yourself in from a hard day of work. The sour cream will keep in your fridge for weeks unopened. Opened, it will keep for about a week. Just give it a stir if it separates.

I pack this to take to work because pasta retains its texture when you heat it up in the microwave.

Cook the pasta according to package directions. While the pasta water comes to a boil, heat the oil in a large frying pan until medium hot. Add the frozen vegetables and stir. Cover the pan to help defrost the vegetables. Stir every couple of minutes until the vegetables are thawed and softened.

When the pasta is done, drain it well and put it in a large bowl. Add the cooked vegetables and sour cream and squeeze the lemon half over all. Add chopped fresh herbs if you have them. Mix and season with salt and pepper. Enjoy!

319 calories | 6.6 g fat | 2.0 g saturated fat
53.2 g carbohydrates | 4.9 g sugar | 16.1 g protein
11.9 g fiber | 68 mg sodium

Airy and Easy Mac and Cheese

**Serves 8,
1 cup per serving**

Nonstick spray

½ pound whole-wheat elbow
macaroni or other cut pasta shape

1 pound frozen cauliflower florets

3 large eggs

4 cups shredded sharp Cheddar
cheese (12 ounces; see Note)

1½ cups whole milk

2 small garlic cloves, minced

1 tablespoon Dijon mustard

¼ teaspoon salt

Macaroni and cheese is a staple in my house. My son would eat this dish for breakfast, lunch, and dinner if I let him. The key to making a healthier version is to use whole-wheat elbow macaroni and cauliflower instead of regular white pasta.

Should you use light cheese for this dish? I think there are a couple of reasons to stick to regular sharp Cheddar for macaroni and cheese. The problem is that reducing the fat from cheese means removing some protein and calcium, too. You don't want to make this dish less nutritious; you just want to make it lighter.

My version takes out half of the pasta and adds a pound of cauliflower to reduce calories and boost nutrition. How does it taste? When I changed from regular pasta to whole grain and cauliflower, my family hardly noticed the difference.

Be careful to keep your serving size in check if you are watching your weight. Macaroni and cheese, even my "airy" version, is still on the "treat" end of the healthy-eating spectrum.

Preheat the oven to 350°F and spray a 3-quart (9 × 13 × 2-inch) casserole dish with nonstick spray.

In a large pot, boil 1 quart water for the pasta. Cook the macaroni for 4 minutes and add the frozen cauliflower. Boil for another 3 minutes and test the macaroni for doneness. When al dente, drain the macaroni and cauliflower and reserve.

In a large bowl, beat the eggs. Mix in the cheese, milk, garlic, mustard, and salt. Add the pasta and cauliflower, mix, and transfer to the casserole dish. Bake until golden and bubbling, about 25 minutes. Enjoy!

Note: You can buy shredded Cheddar cheese or grate it yourself. I use the grater attachment for my food processor to make an easy job of this.

---

337 calories | 17.8 g fat | 10.4 g saturated fat | 27.1 g carbohydrates | 4.1 g sugar | 19.5 g protein
3.8 g fiber | 421 mg sodium

Beef and Veggie Cottage Pie

Serves 8 without mashed potatoes
or puff pastry, 1 ½ cups per
serving; serves 10 with puff
pastry, 1 ¼ cups per serving;
serves 10 with mashed potatoes,
2 cups per serving

Nonstick spray

1 pound 90% lean ground beef

1 large onion, roughly chopped

1 (28-ounce) can low-sodium
diced tomatoes with juice

2 pounds frozen mixed vegetables

2 tablespoons Worcestershire
sauce

1 tablespoon Dijon mustard

1 sheet puff pastry, thawed, or
1 recipe Mashed Potatoes with
Cauliflower (page 207) (optional)

Cottage pie is one of those foods that you see on menus in Irish and English pubs; it pairs well with beer. If you are looking for comfort food, this is a great recipe for you.

The original recipe was created to use up the leftover roast meat and potatoes from the night before. My version uses ground beef because most of us aren't eating beef roasts very often.

The ratio here is 1 pound of meat to 2 pounds of vegetables. Frozen veggie blends, such as corn, carrots, and green beans, are an easy and inexpensive way to add nutrients and fiber to any dish.

There are a couple of different ways to complete this recipe. First, you don't have to add any topping to the filling (or just toss on some bread crumbs).

Second, if you want a real "pie" effect, you can add a big slab of puff pastry for a buttery topping to the dish. Unfortunately, this does add significant calories, but you are still eating a bunch of vegetables mixed in with red meat.

Finally, if you have time, you can add a topping of mashed potatoes. My recipe includes cauliflower so you are getting another big serving of vegetables with this addition.

I like to add ketchup and Tabasco to my portion to make it more spicy and sweet.

If using puff pastry, thaw it in the fridge or on the counter before starting the recipe.

TO MAKE THE FILLING

Preheat the oven to 400°F. Coat a 9 × 13 × 2-inch casserole or several smaller baking dishes with nonstick cooking spray.

Heat a large saucepan over medium-high heat. Cook the beef until brown, stirring frequently. Remove the beef from the pan, drain the fat, and add the onion. Cook the onion until softened, then add the tomatoes with their juice, frozen mixed vegetables, Worcestershire sauce, Dijon mustard, and ½ cup water.

Put the filling in the casserole dish.

FOR "NAKED" COTTAGE PIE

Bake for 50 minutes or until bubbling hot.

---

227 calories | 7.1 g fat | 2.7 g saturated fat | 21.3 g carbohydrates | 7.7 g sugar
19.2 g protein | 6.6 g fiber | 148 mg sodium

FOR "PUFF PASTRY" COTTAGE PIE

Stretch the pastry sheet over the filling, or cut the sheet into squares and dot the filling with pastry. Cook for 50 minutes, or until the pastry is golden brown and the filling is bubbling.

319 calories | 15.1 g fat | 3.5 g saturated fat | 28.3 g carbohydrates | 6.4 g sugar
17.2 g protein | 5.6 g fiber | 180 mg sodium

FOR "MASHED POTATOES" COTTAGE PIE

Spread 6 cups of mashed potatoes evenly over the filling. Bake for 50 minutes, until heated through and the potatoes are slightly browned.

322 calories | 8.8 g fat | 4.0 g saturated fat | 43 g carbohydrates | 8.7 g sugar
19.2 g protein | 8.9 g fiber | 339 mg sodium

Stovetop Tuna Casserole

**Serves 4,
about 1 ½ cups each**

2 (5-ounce) cans chunk white albacore tuna packed in water, drained

1 cup frozen peas

1 cup frozen chopped broccoli

1 cup frozen carrot slices

1 can low-sodium cream of mushroom soup (such as Campbell's)

1 cup whole-wheat elbow macaroni

¼ cup grated Parmesan cheese

Salt and pepper to taste

Tuna casserole is one of those meals that everyone loves. My version is fast, economical, and packed with vegetables. It isn't going to win a James Beard award for culinary excellence, but your kids will eat it without complaining.

I use low-sodium cream of mushroom soup (Campbell's) because the amount of sodium in tuna is fairly high.

Put the tuna, peas, broccoli, carrot slices, soup, and 1 cup water in a large saucepan and bring to a boil. Add the elbow macaroni, reduce the heat to a strong simmer, cover, and cook for 8 minutes, or until the macaroni is tender.

Add the Parmesan cheese and season with salt and pepper.

---

343 calories | 9.8 g fat | 2.9 g saturated fat

40.3 g carbohydrates | 7.7 g sugar | 23.5 g protein

8.1 g fiber | 580 mg sodium

Sneaky Zucchini Lasagna

Serves 8,
1 ¼ cups per serving

1 (15-ounce) container part-skim ricotta cheese

½ cup grated Parmesan cheese

1 large egg

1 (25-ounce) jar tomato sauce, no cheese or sugar added (such as marinara sauce)

1 (14.5-ounce) can diced fire-roasted tomatoes with juice

1 large zucchini, sliced lengthwise into 7 or 8 slices

6 no-bake lasagna noodles

1 cup grated mozzarella cheese

I am not a big fan of adding pureed vegetables to food, but sometimes it's a way to sneak in some veggies without anyone catching on. This recipe hides slices of zucchini under sauce and cheese.

When my kids first tried this recipe, no one noticed they were eating zucchini for half the meal. Then, my eight-year-old found a green edge and demanded to know what it was. I told her it was "green pasta" but she was too smart for that and removed the rest of the zucchini.

If you have super picky eaters, try peeling the zucchini so they don't notice the tell-tale green. My six-year-old son didn't notice the zucchini and ate everything on his plate.

This isn't really cooking. You are just putting the pieces together into a lovely casserole. The recipe is a bit high in sodium because the premade tomato sauce and fire-roasted tomatoes have a lot of added salt. If you are concerned about your sodium level, use low-sodium versions of these products and you will be fine.

One serving of this includes 36 percent of your daily value of calcium and 11 percent of your iron.

To slice the zucchini lengthwise, trim off the stem, then cut carefully down one side to make a flat area so the zucchini won't roll all over the cutting board. Then slice down the length of the squash.

Preheat the oven to 375°F degrees.

Mix the ricotta, Parmesan, and egg in a small bowl. In another bowl, combine the tomato sauce and diced tomatoes.

Pour 1 cup of the tomato mixture into a 9 × 13 × 2-inch casserole. Layer all of the zucchini slices over the sauce.

Dollop half the ricotta mixture over the zucchini and top with another cup of the tomato mixture. Cover with 3 pasta sheets and spread with the rest of the ricotta mixture. Add 1 cup sauce and top with the remaining 3 pasta sheets. Top with the rest of the sauce and cover with grated mozzarella.

Cover with foil and bake for 40 minutes. Remove the foil and bake for another 10 minutes to finish melting the cheese. After taking the lasagna out of the oven, let it sit for 5 to 10 minutes to firm up.

---

254 calories | 10.8 g fat | 5.7 g saturated fat | 24.3 g carbohydrates | 6.3 g sugar
16.6 g protein | 2.5 g fiber | 644 mg sodium

Chicken and Vegetable Potpie

Serves 8,
1 ½ cups per serving

**1 ½ pounds boneless, skinless
chicken breasts**

**2 pounds frozen mixed
vegetables, thawed**

**1 (10-ounce) container Buitoni
Light Alfredo Sauce**

1 teaspoon dried thyme

Black pepper to taste

**½ package refrigerated or
frozen piecrust, thawed to room
temperature**

A normal chicken potpie has top and bottom crusts and is packed with chicken in a creamy sauce. To lighten it, I have added 2 pounds of vegetables and used just a top crust. To give the filling creamy goodness I used Buitoni Light Alfredo Sauce. You can find it nationwide in the fresh pasta section, and it tastes delicious. Even if you are accustomed to very heavy potpie, I don't think you'll miss the fat and calories in this version.

Any packaged piecrust will be fine for this recipe. I store the other half in my freezer for the next potpie night. Or you can double the recipe and have a casserole waiting in the freezer for a hectic night.

You can use 1 ½ pounds of leftover chopped cooked chicken or turkey for this recipe. Be aware that the calorie count will go up if you use dark meat. Just be sure to thaw the mixed vegetables before you add them to the bowl.

Preheat the oven to 350°F.

Cook the chicken breasts according to the recipe for Poached Boneless, Skinless Chicken Breast for Every Day (page 156). About 5 minutes before the chicken is done, add the thawed mixed vegetables.

Drain the chicken and vegetables. Chop the chicken into small pieces and put the vegetables and chicken in a large bowl. Mix in the Alfredo sauce, thyme, and black pepper.

Pour the filling into a 9 × 13 × 2-inch casserole. Cut the piecrust into 8 pieces and lay them on top of the filling, covering as much as you can.

Bake for 40 minutes, or until the crust is browned and the filling is hot.

---

319 calories | 9.8 g fat | 3.9 g saturated fat | 29.3 g carbohydrates | 6.8 g sugar | 28.5 g protein
7.0 g fiber | 651 mg sodium

Mighty Meatloaf

2½ pounds 85% lean
ground beef

1 large egg

¼ cup grated Parmesan cheese

2 tablespoons
Worcestershire sauce

½ cup minced fresh flat-leaf
parsley

1 medium onion, grated

1 large carrot, grated

2 garlic cloves, minced

1 (8-ounce) package presliced
and washed white mushrooms,
chopped

2 teaspoons dried thyme

½ cup whole-wheat bread crumbs

Meatloaf, an American classic, usually contains pork, beef, bacon, and maybe even veal. While I love the stuff, it is easy to make it healthier without too many people noticing.

This is a recipe for a food processor if you have one. I use the chopper attachment to make my bread crumbs and chop my garlic and mushrooms. I use the grater attachment for the onion and carrot. This saves a huge amount of time.

I was unable to find whole-wheat bread crumbs in my local store. To make your own, tear a slice of whole-wheat bread into small pieces and whirl them in a food processor or blender. If you have neither of these devices, just use a knife and mince the bread into the smallest pieces possible.

I used 85% lean ground beef because it is affordable, but it has more fat per serving than leaner cuts. Be sure to measure your 4-ounce serving to ensure the correct portion size. This recipe makes a lot; you can freeze leftovers for future meals.

Preheat the oven to 375°F.

In a large bowl, combine all ingredients and mix well. Divide the mixture in half and pat into two 4½ × 8½-inch (1½-quart) loaf pans. Bake for 55 to 60 minutes, until an instant-read thermometer inserted in the center reads 160°F.

---

217 calories | 12.6 g fat | 4.8 g saturated fat | 3.2 g carbohydrates | 1.4 g sugar
21.5 g protein | 0.7 g fiber | 121 mg sodium

Sides

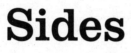

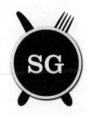

Roasted Vegetables

Why would I devote an entire section of this book to roasted vegetables? Because they will change your life. They are low calorie, versatile, and nutritious, and require very little preparation time.

All you need is a sharp knife, a cutting board, rimmed baking sheets, and an oven and you have the tools for making these recipes. A couple of suggestions:

1. **Buy vegetables that are in season.** They will be fresher and less expensive.

2. **Prepare them as soon as you get home from the store.** Make roasting vegetables part of putting away your groceries.

3. **Put them in everything**—salads, omelets, sandwiches, casseroles, quesadillas, you name it.

I have included a recipe for slow cooker caramelized onions in this section because it is essentially the same as roasting, just with a different piece of equipment.

At the end of this section are two suggestions on how to create a larger meal with your roasted vegetables. Using pasta, tortillas, and cheese, you can make something super fast and healthy.

Crunchy Sweet Roasted Broccoli

**Serves 8,
4 ounces per serving**

---

2 pounds broccoli crowns

**2 tablespoons extra-virgin
olive oil**

1 teaspoon sugar

½ teaspoon salt

**Freshly ground black pepper
to taste (optional)**

What if you could make broccoli taste as good as, say, potato chips? Would you give that recipe a try? This roasted broccoli recipe is one of the favorites on Snack-Girl.com because it convinces even die-hard broccoli haters to give this vegetable another chance.

It is super easy to make and has a secret ingredient (sugar) that helps soften broccoli's slightly bitter edge. I usually make a couple of trays of this and store it in the fridge to add to salads, lunches, and omelets and put straight into my mouth.

Position an oven rack in the lowest position and preheat the oven to 500°F. Line a large rimmed baking sheet with aluminum foil (for easy cleanup). Place the prepared sheet on the lowest oven rack while the oven heats.

Cut the broccoli crowns into 4 wedges, cutting lengthwise from the crown through the stem. Place the broccoli in a large bowl and drizzle with the olive oil. Sprinkle the sugar, salt, and optional pepper over the broccoli and toss to combine.

When the oven is hot, transfer the broccoli to the baking sheet and roast until slightly browned and very crunchy, about 15 minutes.

---

64 calories | 3.9 g fat | 0.5 g saturated fat | 6.5 g carbohydrates
2.5 g sugar | 3.4 g protein | 3.0 g fiber | 178 mg sodium

Roasted Brussels Sprouts

**Serves 4,
4 ounces per serving**

---

1 pound fresh Brussels sprouts

2 tablespoons extra-virgin olive oil

Salt and pepper to taste

This recipe was a game changer for me. My dad boiled Brussels sprouts into smelly, mushy, ugly blobs. No wonder I used to hate Brussels sprouts; now I love them.

When you roast Brussels sprouts the natural sugars caramelize, and all of a sudden you have a different food altogether. Instead of a mushy blob, you have a crunchy side dish that will change your life. Really.

One important tip—do not buy Brussels sprouts and leave them in your refrigerator for a week. This is an excellent way to ensure that they taste terrible. The fresher the Brussels sprouts, the sweeter they will taste.

You can serve this recipe cold, room temperature, or hot. These would make a great party snack with some toothpicks and mustard dipping sauce on the side.

This recipe will not work with frozen Brussels sprouts. Make it in the fall or winter, when you can find fresh Brussels sprouts.

Heat the oven to 400°F. Line a rimmed baking sheet with aluminum foil (for easy cleanup).

Cut off the ends of the sprouts, remove any loose leaves, and cut in half. Place the sprouts on the baking sheet and, using your hands, toss with the olive oil, salt, and pepper. Roast until browned or a bit blackened, 30 to 40 minutes.

---

109 calories | 7.3 g fat | 1.1 g saturated fat | 10.2 g carbohydrates | 2.5 g sugar | 3.8 g protein
4.3 g fiber | 28 mg sodium

Roasted Asparagus

**Serves 4,
4 ounces per serving**

**1 bunch asparagus
(about 1 pound)**

**1 tablespoon extra-virgin
olive oil**

Salt and pepper to taste

**Grated Parmesan cheese
(optional)**

**Lemon wedges
(optional)**

Fresh spring asparagus is an invitation to dance in the streets to welcome the end of winter. When I see local asparagus in the store I know it's time to dig my sandals out of my closet.

There is nothing to fear about buying or cooking asparagus. A few tips:

• Look for the thicker stalks—most chefs think they taste better.

• Use them the day you buy them—aging them in your fridge is not a good idea.

• Do not boil—yuck!

You can wrap asparagus in thin slices of ham or prosciutto for a nice party snack.

I sprinkle asparagus with grated Parmesan cheese (just a little) to add a salty, cheesy element. Or skip the cheese and squeeze fresh lemon juice over the stalks.

Roast a couple of bunches of asparagus and keep them in your fridge for snacking. Add them to salads or omelets. My kids eat these because we call them "trees" and they pretend they are dinosaurs.

Preheat the oven to 400°F. Line a rimmed baking sheet with aluminum foil (for easy cleanup). Snap off the tough ends of the asparagus and discard. Toss the asparagus with the olive oil, salt, and pepper. Cook for 15 minutes (or until desired tenderness). Sprinkle with Parmesan cheese or lemon juice and serve immediately or refrigerate, tightly covered, for up to a week.

WITHOUT PARMESAN CHEESE OR LEMON

53 calories | 3.6 g fat | 0.6 g saturated fat | 4.4 g carbohydrates | 2.1 g sugar

2.5 g protein | 2.4 g fiber | 2 mg sodium

Roasted Cauliflower

**Serves 4,
1 cup per serving**

**8 cups fresh cauliflower (1 large
head) or 2 pounds frozen
cauliflower**

2 tablespoons soy sauce

1 tablespoon canola oil

1 teaspoon sugar

**½ teaspoon black pepper
(optional)**

Cauliflower is one of the foods you should make the effort to eat (if you can stand it): A cup has a mere 28 calories, plus 92 percent of your daily value of vitamin C. However, I will admit that nothing is more boring than steamed or boiled cauliflower.

This recipe requires a bit of marinating for the cauliflower to shine but if you don't have time, just skip this step. I have included directions for frozen cauliflower. It will take longer and won't be as crisp as fresh cauliflower, but it is still tasty.

Be careful with soy sauce—a single tablespoon has 900 milligrams of sodium. The sodium in this recipe is on the high side, so skip the soy sauce and use a little salt if this is a concern.

Preheat the oven to 450°F. Line a rimmed baking sheet with aluminum foil (for easy cleanup).

Chop the fresh cauliflower into small florets. (If using frozen cauliflower, thaw it in the microwave and then dry it off with paper towels.)

Combine the soy sauce, canola oil, sugar, and pepper (if using) in a large bowl. Add the cauliflower and marinate for 20 minutes, mixing once. Spread the cauliflower out on the lined baking sheet. Roast for 15 to 20 minutes for fresh cauliflower or 30 minutes for frozen cauliflower, until browned.

Serve hot, cold, or at room temperature.

88 calories | 3.6 g fat | 0.7 g saturated fat | 12.3 g carbohydrates | 6.0 g sugar
4.5 g protein | 5.1 g fiber | 511 mg sodium

Roasted Acorn Squash

Serves 4,
½ pound per serving

2 medium acorn squash
(about 1 pound each)

2 tablespoons butter

2 tablespoons light or
dark brown sugar
(or maple syrup)

Salt and pepper to taste

Squash is an inexpensive, easy-to-cook nutritional powerhouse.

Acorn, butternut, delicata, spaghetti, calabaza, and kabocha are squash varieties that I can pick up for a dollar per pound or less from my local farmers during the fall.

An *entire* medium acorn squash (without butter) will set you back only 172 calories, and you get 32 percent of your daily value of vitamin A, 17 percent of your iron, and 79 percent of your vitamin C.

However, Snack Girl must confess to a certain dislike of squash. I have tried steamed squash with nothing on it and find it tasteless. If you add a wee bit of butter and sugar, you infuse it with some flavor and all of a sudden it becomes addictive.

Are you ruining its nutritive properties with a little fat? No, you are simply making it palatable so you can enjoy it and get all those nutrients in your body working for you. Fat actually helps you absorb nutrients in vegetables, so don't be afraid to add a little.

Preheat the oven to 400°F. Cut the squash in half and scoop out the seeds (see Note). Soften the butter in the microwave, mix it with the sugar or syrup, and brush the inside of the squash with the mixture. Add salt and pepper to taste. Place the squash on a rimmed baking sheet cut side up and roast for 1 hour, or until tender. Serve hot or at room temperature. Enjoy!

Note: If you like roasted seeds, you can roast the squash seeds alongside your squash. Remove the strings from the seeds and dry them with a paper towel. Add about 1 tablespoon olive oil for a cup of seeds and salt and pepper to taste. Spread on a rimmed baking sheet lined with foil and roast for about 20 minutes, or until golden brown. Toss the seeds after about 10 minutes to help them cook evenly.

154 calories | 6.0 g fat | 3.7 g saturated fat | 26.9 g carbohydrates | 4.4 g sugar
1.8 g protein | 3.2 g fiber | 49 mg sodium

FOR 2 TABLESPOONS ROASTED SQUASH SEEDS WITHOUT ADDED SALT
142 calories | 12.4 g fat | 1.9 g saturated fat | 2.7 g carbohydrates | 0 g sugar
5.3 g protein | 0.7 g fiber | 3 mg sodium

Roasted Mushrooms

Serves 4,
½ cup per serving

---

1 pound white mushrooms,
wiped clean

2 tablespoons extra-virgin
olive oil

These are brilliant. They are packed with flavor and, if you don't mind cleaning mushrooms properly, easy to cook.

Mushrooms should not be rinsed in water because they tend to soak it up like a sponge. I take a wet paper towel and carefully wipe off the dirt until they are clean. Yes, it is a pain, but these mushrooms are such a great addition to salads, omelets, quesadillas, pasta, whatever, that I keep making them.

They are also very high in iron, niacin, potassium, and vitamin B_6. You can't lose.

Preheat the oven to 475°F. Line a rimmed baking sheet with parchment paper.

Trim the mushroom stems to remove any rough sections. Wipe any dirt from the mushrooms with a damp paper towel. Put the mushrooms on the baking sheet and drizzle with the oil. Roast the mushrooms for 15 minutes, remove from the oven, and toss. Roast for another 15 minutes, or until deep brown and firm.

---

84 calories | 7.3 g fat | 1.0 g saturated fat

3.7 g carbohydrates | 1.9 g sugar | 3.6 g protein

1.1 g fiber | 6 mg sodium

Slow Cooker Caramelized Onions

**Serves 8,
¼ cup per serving**

3 pounds yellow onions

Nonstick spray

2 tablespoons extra-virgin
olive oil

Caramelized onions are one of those amazing foods that can transform a mundane dish into something special. I have hated cooking them because they take forever on the stove (and you have to keep your eye on them). The slow cooker is the solution to having caramelized onions without the work.

Use them like a condiment to give flavor to all sorts of meals, such as pizza, omelets, baked potatoes, salads, soups, dips—you get the idea. You could even add some to your oatmeal with a dash of soy sauce. The only limit to their uses is your imagination.

Cut the onions in half and peel off the rough skin. Cut into ¼-inch slices. Coat the inside of a 6-quart slow cooker with cooking spray. Add the onions and olive oil and separate all the onion slices into individual rings using a fork, tongs, or your hands.

Cover and cook on high for 7 hours. They should be dark brown; if they start to burn at the edges of the slow cooker, give them a stir.

Pack these up in small containers and freeze for later use.

98 calories | 3.7 g fat | 0.6 g saturated fat | 15.9 g carbohydrates
7.2 g sugar | 1.9 g protein | 2.9 g fiber | 7 mg sodium

Roasted Vegetables with Pasta

Serves 1

1 serving of Crunchy Sweet Roasted Broccoli (page 193) or other roasted vegetable from this section

½ cup cooked whole-wheat penne

2 tablespoons pasta water

2 tablespoons grated Parmesan cheese

Pasta, such as elbow macaroni, shells, spirals, wagon wheels, and ziti, doubles in size when it cooks, so you need ¼ cup dried to get ½ cup cooked. Keep in mind that ½ cup cooked pasta has about 100 calories and 2 tablespoons of grated Parmesan, just over 50 calories.

When you cook the pasta, scoop out some of the water with a ladle before you drain it. This pasta water is flavorful and gives the dish more moisture without adding any calories (though depending on how much salt you use in the pasta water, it will add some sodium).

Make this light meal with any of the delicious roasted vegetables in this section. It is also an easy lunch that you can toss together and take to work.

Mix the vegetables, pasta, cooking water, and Parmesan cheese together in a medium bowl and heat in the microwave until hot (about 2 minutes).

---

287 calories | 12.1 g fat | 3.2 g saturated fat

34.3 g carbohydrates | 6.0 g sugar | 15.1 g protein | 8.4 g fiber

258 mg sodium

Roasted Vegetable Quesadilla

½ medium Roasted Acorn
Squash (page 200)
or 1 serving of another roasted
vegetable from this section

2 tablespoons grated sharp
Cheddar cheese

1 large whole-wheat tortilla

Fresh salsa
(optional)

This is another quick meal that you can make when you have roasted vegetables in your refrigerator.

A large whole-wheat tortilla has about 110 calories, and 2 tablespoons of grated Cheddar cheese has 60, so keep that in mind if you create this with another roasted vegetable.

I like to make this quesadilla with roasted squash because I can use just a little cheese and still get a soft layer of yumminess inside the tortilla. Quesadillas are usually packed with cheese; this healthier version is packed with vegetables.

Serve it with salsa, just like the real thing.

Mash the squash in a small bowl with a fork. Spread it on half the tortilla and top with grated cheese. Fold over the other half, making a half circle.

Heat a frying pan over medium heat and toast the tortilla until the cheese melts. Serve immediately with salsa or plain.

WITHOUT SALSA

321 calories | 11.6 g fat | 6.7 g saturated fat

49.1 g carbohydrates | 4.4 g sugar | 9.3 g protein

6.2 g fiber | 266 mg sodium

Mashed Potatoes, Fries, Beans, and Rice

Mashed Potatoes with Cauliflower

Serves 12,
½ cup per serving

**4 large red potatoes
(about 2 pounds)**

1 pound frozen cauliflower

2 tablespoons butter

2 tablespoons sour cream

¾ teaspoon salt

Who doesn't like mashed potatoes? They are the ultimate comfort food. And you will be amazed at how little butter or cream you need to make mashed potatoes sing.

Sneak in a lighter ingredient to increase the volume and decrease the calories. Cooked cauliflower has only 28 calories per cup versus boiled potatoes (134 calories per cup).

I choose not to peel my potatoes because I am lazy. I use red potatoes, which are easy to wash, slice, and mash. If you don't have a potato masher, you should get one. Not only is it fun to mash your own potatoes, it's also good exercise!

Scrub the potatoes and cut into 1-inch chunks. Put the potatoes in a large stockpot with water to cover by about ½ inch. Bring to a boil and cook at a medium boil for 15 minutes, or until the potatoes yield to a fork. Add the cauliflower to the pot with the potatoes and cook for 5 minutes.

Drain the vegetables and mash with a potato masher. Add the butter, sour cream, and salt. Mix well and serve.

117 calories | 2.5 g fat | 1.5 g saturated fat
21.6 g carbohydrates | 2.1 g sugar | 3.1 g protein
3.0 g fiber | 181 mg sodium

Homemade Skinny Fries

Serves 4,
4 ounces per serving

---

1 pound russet potatoes

1 tablespoon extra-virgin olive oil

Salt and pepper to taste

So, this isn't the simplest recipe: Making homemade "fries" means slicing potatoes into thin strips, soaking and drying them, and then roasting them for 30 to 40 minutes.

What will you get for all your work? You can enjoy fries without guilt.

Soaking the potatoes in cold water leaches out some of the starch, making the fries crisper, so don't skip this step. I leave the skin on because I like the flavor and texture. Feel free to remove it if you don't like it.

I use parchment paper in this recipe instead of aluminum foil because I found that the fries stuck to the foil. Parchment paper works like a charm and will cost you about $3 for a roll. I love the stuff.

Preheat the oven to 425°F. Line a rimmed baking sheet with parchment paper. Fill a large bowl with ice water.

Scrub the potatoes and cut them lengthwise into strips ¼ inch wide and 2 to 3 inches long. Place them in the ice water and let soak for 10 minutes. Rinse with cold water and dry with paper towels.

Put the potatoes on the baking sheet in a single layer, drizzle them with olive oil, and dust with salt and pepper. Roast for 15 minutes and take out of the oven. Turn them over and roast for another 15 to 20 minutes. If you like really crispy fries, bake an additional 8 minutes. Serve immediately.

---

108 calories | 3.6 g fat | 0.5 g saturated fat | 17.8 g carbohydrates | 1.3 g sugar | 1.9 g protein
2.7 g fiber | 7 mg sodium

Slow Cooker Red Kidney Beans

**Makes 7 cups,
½ cup per serving**

---

1 pound dried red kidney beans

1 smoked ham hock (8 to 12 ounces)

1 onion, chopped

1 teaspoon ground cumin

2 teaspoons smoked paprika

2 teaspoons salt or to taste

Did you know that the slow cooker was originally a dried bean cooker? Yes, this great invention came out of the need to cook dried beans for hours to make them edible.

Dried beans are incredibly inexpensive; they taste better and are lower in sodium than canned beans.

This recipe will work for any dried bean except lentils or split peas (which take far less time to cook). I use a ham hock to add some depth of flavor. Yes, this adds fat, but beans taste better with fat, plus you get 15 percent of your daily value of iron and almost 12 grams of protein in every serving. The key here is that the meat is a flavoring agent, not the focus of the dish. Feel free to add your favorite spices to make these beans work for you.

These beans store well in the freezer and are great with rice, salsa, or tortillas or just served in a bowl with a little cheese on top. You can also add these to soups, such as Mexican Chicken Soup (page 169), for bulk and additional protein and fiber.

Wash the beans and soak overnight in a large bowl of cold water. They will swell up, so ensure there is plenty of space. Drain the beans and put in a 4- or 6-quart slow cooker.

Add the ham hock, onion, and 1 quart water. Cook on high for 3½ to 4 hours, until the beans are tender.

Remove the ham hock from the pot and take off the skin and bone. Chop up any ham you find and put it back in the slow cooker with the beans.

Season the beans with cumin, smoked paprika, and salt.

---

165 calories | 4.2 g fat | 1.5 g saturated fat | 20.8 g carbohydrates | 1.0 g sugar

11.0 g protein | 5.2 g fiber | 354 mg sodium

Easy Baked Brown Rice

**Makes 6 cups,
½ cup per serving**

---

3 cups brown rice

2 tablespoons unsalted butter

**1 teaspoon coarse salt
(or ½ teaspoon fine salt)**

The main difference between white rice and brown rice is the processing. When only the outermost layer of a grain of rice (the husk) is removed, brown rice is produced. To produce white rice the bran and germ layer are removed, leaving mostly the starchy endosperm.

The processing that converts brown rice into white destroys 67 percent of the vitamin B_3, 80 percent of the vitamin B_1, 90 percent of the vitamin B_6, half of the manganese, half of the phosphorus, 60 percent of the iron, and all of the dietary fiber and essential fatty acids. Fully milled and polished white rice is required to be "enriched" with vitamins B_1, B_3, and iron.

You don't want to lose all those nutrients, do you? But white rice is so easy to cook and eat (which is why we love it so).

Does brown rice taste like cardboard? It does take a little getting used to—but you might start to crave its nutty flavor. I add a little butter for flavor as well. If you think you will hate it, try mixing cooked white rice with your cooked brown rice to start. Then, slowly, use just brown rice.

This technique is my favorite: It allows me to easily cook a ton of rice with hardly any stirring, and no watching the pot. *And* the pot is super easy to clean, with no burnt caked-on rice to scrub off!

Eat it for breakfast mixed with raisins and nuts, add it to your packed lunch, or make a rice salad or fried rice with it.

Preheat the oven to 375°F. In a teakettle or pot, bring 5 cups water to a boil. Put the rice in a 9 × 13 × 2-inch casserole or other baking dish that will hold at least 12 cups; if the dish does not have a lid, use aluminum foil to cover it. Dot the butter into the rice and sprinkle on the salt.

Add the boiling water, stir, cover, and bake for 1 hour. After 1 hour, remove the cover and fluff the rice with a fork.

Serve or put in containers to freeze for later use.

---

126 calories | 2.7 g fat | 1.4 g saturated fat | 22.9 g carbohydrates | 2.3 g protein
1.8 g fiber | 179 mg sodium

Faster-Than-White-Rice Cauliflower Rice

**Makes 8 cups,
1 cup per serving**

_____

1 head cauliflower

Have you ever measured how much rice comes in one of those take-out containers from the Chinese place?

I am not advocating for a low-carb diet but I am pointing out that a cup of white rice has around 200 calories (without adding butter). Rice is ridiculously easy to eat without noticing how much you have consumed.

Cauliflower has 28 calories for an entire cup. You can mix it into regular rice and cut your calories by quite a lot while increasing your vegetable consumption. It's a win-win.

Fortunately, making "cauliflower rice" is almost as easy as making regular rice. All you do is grate a cauliflower into a bowl and microwave it! If you don't own a microwave, you can steam the cauliflower on the stove with ½ cup water in a covered pot for 5 to 6 minutes. Just drain it when it is done.

I substitute cauliflower rice in my favorite rice dishes. For example, I add some canned beans (drained and rinsed), salsa, and a little cheese and heat it up for a fast lunch.

Grate or chop the cauliflower into pieces the size of rice kernels. Use the grater attachment on the food processor, if you have one—it is the quickest and easiest way to get the cauliflower small enough. Heat the cauliflower in a microwave-safe bowl on high for 3 minutes and stir. Repeat until tender (6 to 8 minutes).

Refrigerate for up to 1 week.

---

28 calories | 0.6 g fat | 0 g saturated fat | 5.0 g carbohydrates | 2.4 g sugar | 2.2 g protein

2.8 g fiber | 18 mg sodium

Snacks

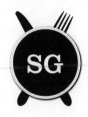

Snack Girl is famous for her snacks (duh). Over the years, I have developed a bunch of easy options to help my readers dodge the junk food temptations that surround us. These snacks will work as meals if you mix and match a few together or triple the portions. When I am in a hurry (and no one is looking), this is how I eat.

The key to a healthy snack is to keep the calories to 100 to 200 per portion and pack in as much nutrition as you can. My favorite snack (drum roll please) is apple slices spread with some natural peanut butter. I love that it is salty, sweet, crunchy, and creamy and I feel full after I eat it. An apple and peanut butter is a better snack versus just an apple because the peanut butter adds fat and protein to keep you going. It is simple and if you carry a pocketknife, you can make it on the go.

This snack section has two parts. The first is a list of some of the easiest, fastest, most nutritious snacks in the West (and the East, North, and South). The second is a group of recipes that take a little more time to prepare, but are worth it. I have included three recipes for kale because it is so nutritious and I want to convert you into a kale lover.

10 Sweet Snacks

Apples and Peanut Butter

Core and quarter a medium apple (3-inch diameter). Spread with 2 teaspoons of creamy natural peanut butter or almond butter.

---

147 calories | 5.3 g fat | 0.8 g saturated fat | 24.0 g carbohydrates | 16.3 g sugar | 3.3 g protein
5.7 g fiber | 35 mg sodium

Banana, Peanut Butter, and Raisins

Slice a ripe banana lengthwise and spread with 2 teaspoons of creamy natural peanut butter or almond butter. Dot the top with 5 raisins.

199 calories | 5.8 g fat | 1.0 g saturated fat | 36.1 g carbohydrates | 20.1 g sugar | 3.9 g protein | 4.1 g fiber | 37 mg sodium

Carrot, Cream Cheese, and Raisin Wrap

Grate 1 small carrot. Spread 1 tablespoon cream cheese on a 100 percent whole-wheat tortilla. Add grated carrots and 10 raisins and roll up into a tube. Slice into 10 pieces crosswise.

Serves 2, 5 pieces per serving

112 calories | 2.4 g fat | 1.1 g saturated fat | 21.2 g carbohydrates | 6.8 g sugar | 3.0 g protein | 2.7 g fiber | 102 mg sodium

Yogurt with Jam

Mix 4 ounces (½ cup) plain whole-milk yogurt with 1½ teaspoons of your favorite jam.

123 calories | 4.0 g fat | 2.3 g saturated fat | 16.3 g carbohydrates | 7.0 g sugar | 5.0 g protein | 0 g fiber | 80 mg sodium

Cantaloupe Bowl with Blueberries and Yogurt

Cut the cantaloupe in half and spoon out the seeds. Cover the remaining half with plastic wrap and store in the fridge for another use (or another snack.) Spoon ½ cup plain yogurt into the hollow. Top with 10 fresh blueberries.

---

129 calories | 4.2 g fat | 2.5 g saturated fat | 16.9 g carbohydrates | 14.0 g sugar
7.3 g protein | 1.5 g fiber | 64 mg sodium

Cottage Cheese, Raisins, and Cinnamon

Add 10 raisins and ¼ teaspoon cinnamon to ½ cup low-fat cottage cheese (2% milk fat).

---

156 calories | 2.3 g fat | 1.4 g saturated fat | 18.5 g carbohydrates | 11.1 g sugar
16.1 g protein | 0.7 g fiber | 461 mg sodium

Chocolate Smoothie

Combine ½ cup whole milk, ½ ripe banana, 1 tablespoon unsweetened cocoa, and 5 ice cubes in a blender. Blend until smooth.

---

138 calories | 4.9 g fat | 1.4 g saturated fat | 21.9 g carbohydrates | 13.7 g sugar
5.6 g protein | 3.3 g fiber | 51 mg sodium

Pumpkin Pie Smoothie

Combine ½ cup canned pumpkin, ¼ cup plain yogurt, 1 teaspoon pumpkin pie spice, ½ banana, 4 ice cubes, and 2 teaspoons maple syrup or honey in a blender. Blend until smooth.

---

160 calories | 1.4 g fat | 0.9 g saturated fat | 33.1 g carbohydrates | 19.6 g sugar | 5.5 g protein
5.3 g fiber | 51 mg sodium

Dried Figs Dipped in Chocolate

Lay a piece of wax paper on a plate. Heat ½ ounce of dark chocolate until melted in the microwave. Dip 5 dried figs into the chocolate, covering only half of the fig. Put on the wax paper–lined plate and sprinkle with a little salt (optional). Refrigerate for 30 minutes.

Serves 5, 1 fig per serving

---

63 calories | 1.0 g fat | 0.6 g saturated fat | 13.8 g carbohydrates | 10.6 g sugar | 0.9 g protein
2.0 g fiber | 4 mg sodium

Sweet Potato Pudding

Mash ½ baked sweet potato (about 4 ounces) in a bowl and mix in ¼ teaspoon cinnamon. Top with ¼ cup low-fat vanilla-flavored yogurt.

---

94 calories | 0.6 g fat | 0.4 g saturated fat | 19.1 g carbohydrates | 10.7 g sugar | 3.4 g protein
1.9 g fiber | 55 mg sodium

10 Savory Snacks

Cheese and Tomato Cracker

Preheat the broiler to high and put 2 Wasa crackers on a baking sheet. Top with 4 slices of fresh tomato, then 4 thin slices of Cheddar cheese (1 ounce). Broil until the cheese is melted.

---

195 calories | 9.7 g fat | 6.0 g saturated fat | 14.0 g carbohydrates | 1.7 g sugar | 9.2 g protein
3.8 g fiber | 179 mg sodium

English Muffin Pizza

Preheat the broiler to high. Spoon 2 tablespoons pizza sauce and ½ ounce grated mozzarella onto half of a 100 percent whole-wheat English muffin. Broil until the cheese is hot and bubbling.

---

128 calories | 3.7 g fat | 2.0 g saturated fat | 17.5 g carbohydrates | 3.8 g sugar | 7.1 g protein
2.7 g fiber | 401 mg sodium

Mini Triscuit Pizzas

Preheat the broiler to high. Place 5 Triscuits on a small baking sheet and top with 2 tablespoons pizza sauce and ½ ounce grated mozzarella. Broil until the cheese is hot and bubbling.

---

180 calories | 7.0 g fat | 2.4 g saturated fat | 24.1 g carbohydrates | 1.1 g sugar | 7.2 g protein
3.5 g fiber | 370 mg sodium

Portobello Mushrooms, Tomatoes, and Mozzarella

Preheat the oven to 350°F. Clean 4 portobello mushroom caps with a damp paper towel and remove the stems. Spoon 1 tablespoon drained canned diced fire-roasted tomatoes into the gills section of each cap. Top each mushroom with 1 ounce grated mozzarella cheese. Bake for 20 minutes, or until the cheese is bubbling.

Serves 4, 1 mushroom per serving

---

123 calories | 5.8 g fat | 3.6 g saturated fat | 8.5 g carbohydrates | 3.2 g sugar | 10.0 g protein
1.8 g fiber | 255 mg sodium

Spicy Roasted Chickpeas

Preheat the oven to 450°F. Drain and rinse one 15-ounce can of chickpeas (garbanzo beans). Mix the chickpeas, 1 tablespoon extra-virgin olive oil, and ½ teaspoon cayenne pepper in a bowl. Spread the chickpeas out on a rimmed baking sheet and bake for 15 minutes. Take out of the oven, shake the pan to ensure the chickpeas brown evenly, and roast for 15 more minutes, until brown and crunchy.

Serves 4, ½ cup per serving

174 calories | 4.9 g fat | 0.7 g saturated fat | 27.3 g carbohydrates | 0 g sugar | 6.0 g protein
5.3 g fiber | 359 mg sodium

Cucumber and French Onion Cheese Wedge

Peel ½ cucumber and cut 10 slices about ¼ inch thick. Spread 1 wedge of Laughing Cow French Onion Cheese onto the slices. Dust with paprika.

58 calories | 2.2 g fat | 1.1 g saturated fat | 6.5 g carbohydrates | 3.5 g sugar | 3.5 g protein
0.8 g fiber | 263 mg sodium

Celery, Whipped Cream Cheese, and Chili Powder

Cut four 3-inch pieces of celery. Fill each stalk with 1 tablespoon whipped cream cheese and dust with chili powder.

131 calories | 10.1 g fat | 6.0 g saturated fat | 6.0 g carbohydrates | 3.2 g sugar | 2.5 g protein
1.1 g fiber | 244 mg sodium

Avocado Toast

Toast 1 slice of 100 percent whole-wheat bread. Spread with ¼ cup ripe avocado and sprinkle with salt to taste.

---

148 calories | 6.3 g fat | 0.8 g saturated fat | 23.1 g carbohydrates | 3.2 g sugar | 4.7 g protein
5.5 g fiber | 203 mg sodium

Celery, Carrot, and Hummus

Peel 1 medium carrot and cut into sticks. Cut one celery stalk into sticks. Serve with ¼ cup prepared hummus or make your own (page 245).

---

135 calories | 6.2 g fat | 0.9 g saturated fat | 16.0 g carbohydrates | 3.6 g sugar | 5.8 g protein
6.1 g fiber | 311 mg sodium

Hard-Boiled Eggs, Roasted Red Pepper, Dijon Mustard, and Mayonnaise

Peel 8 hard-boiled eggs, slice in half, and remove the yolks. Dice ¼ cup roasted red pepper and put in a small bowl with the egg yolks, 2 tablespoons Dijon mustard, and 1 tablespoon mayonnaise. Mix well. Spoon the mixture back into the egg whites and serve.

Serves 4, 4 egg halves per serving

---

148 calories | 10.3 g fat | 2.9 g saturated fat | 2.7 g carbohydrates | 1.5 g sugar | 11.5 g protein
0 g fiber | 265 mg sodium

Kale and Other Healthy Snacks

Crunchy Kale Chips

Serves 3,
⅓ pound per serving

---

1 bunch fresh kale
(about 1 pound)

1 tablespoon extra-virgin
olive oil

Salt to taste

If the green smoothie (page 232) doesn't change your mind about kale, try these. My eight-year-old will just keep shoving these into her mouth. I find myself smiling as I think of all the nutrients she is inhaling.

Why are these so great? Somehow, the roasting tempers kale's bitterness, which can be off-putting. You get these crunchy green chips that are addictive and, for once, addiction is a good thing.

These taste best right out of the oven. If they wait around too long they tend to get soggy. Serve them when you are craving potato chips.

How do you stop eating them? I say, you don't. If you went crazy and ate an entire pound you would have consumed 43 percent of your daily value of iron, 61 percent of your calcium, 1,395 percent of your vitamin A, and only 347 calories.

Compare the 347 calories in kale chips to the 2,560 calories you would have eaten in a pound of potato chips, and you have no problem justifying eating them all.

These chips taste great with a variety of flavors added, such as ground black pepper, curry, or chili powder.

Preheat the oven to 375°F. Line two rimmed baking sheets with parchment paper or aluminum foil (for easy cleanup). Rinse the kale and tear the leaves off the thick stems into chip-size pieces. An easy way to do this is to fold the leaf in half lengthwise and just rip toward the stem. Dry the kale well with paper towels to ensure that it will crisp versus steam.

Divide the kale between the baking sheets and drizzle with olive oil. Dust with salt.

Bake for 15 minutes or until the edges are brown and the kale is crispy when moved in the pan. Enjoy immediately.

116 calories | 5.7 g fat | 0.8 g saturated fat | 15.1 g carbohydrates | 0 g sugar
5.0 g protein | 3.0 g fiber | 65 mg sodium

Massaged Raw Kale Salad

**Serves 4,
1 cup per serving**

**1 bunch fresh kale
(1 pound)**

**2 tablespoons extra-virgin
olive oil**

½ teaspoon salt

**Fresh lemon juice or vinegar
to taste (optional)**

Turn the lights down low and crank up the Barry White. It is time to massage some . . . kale!

I know what you are thinking. Seriously? You want me to massage kale? Hey, I don't even have time to massage my feet. A couple of minutes of foot massage should be an important part of your day and if you get a chance, your kale could use some love too.

Why massage kale? Raw kale by itself is tough and hard to chew. If you chop it small enough and massage it with olive oil, it transforms into a delicious salad. Also, it is a nice treatment for your clean hands, especially in the winter months when skin tends to get dry.

One great reason to use kale for your salad is that it keeps much longer in your fridge than delicate lettuces. It doesn't dissolve into a slimy mess after a few days. Kale is tough.

After you finish massaging the kale, add your favorite salad toppings such as cherry tomatoes, sliced carrots, sliced peppers, or sunflower seeds.

Wash the kale and strip the leaves from the tough stems. Chop with a kitchen knife into small pieces. You will create approximately 4 cups of chopped kale. Dry in a salad spinner. Combine the kale, oil, and salt in a large bowl. Massage the kale with olive oil for 2 minutes or until it reduces in volume. Taste it and add lemon juice or vinegar as needed.

---

117 calories | 7.8 g fat | 1.1 g saturated fat | 11.3 g carbohydrates | 0 g sugar
3.7 g protein | 2.3 g fiber | 339 mg sodium

A Green Smoothie That Doesn't Taste Like Grass

**Serves 1,
2 cups per serving**

1 cup frozen mixed berries

1 cup loosely packed fresh kale leaves, stems torn off

½ banana

I was very suspicious of any smoothie that looked green. You know how Kermit says, "It's not easy being green"? For me, the saying would be "It's not easy *drinking* green"—unless it is a green apple martini, in which case I have the opposite problem.

I made the mistake of planting kale in my garden because it grows well where I live. I was inundated with kale. What was I going to do with all of it? The idea to put it in my blender came from a reader who made smoothies with kale.

This recipe works best with a conventional blender (but not the $15 ones). My blender cost about $50 and it is powerful enough to chop up the kale.

What is amazing to me about this smoothie is that you don't taste the kale. It tastes like a banana-berry concoction that happens to be green! You can also use fresh spinach leaves for the same effect.

Amazingly, my kids drink this and ask for more.

Put the berries, kale, banana, and 1 cup water in a blender and blend until smooth. Enjoy!

156 calories | 1.2 g fat | 0 g saturated fat
37.2 g carbohydrates | 17.3 g sugar | 3.8 g protein
7.9 g fiber | 37 mg sodium

Apple Chips

Serves 4,
½ cup per serving

2 large apples, unpeeled

1 tablespoon sugar

2 teaspoons cinnamon

This is one of those snacks that is incredibly popular on the website because it is so easy and fun to make. The only catch is that you have to wait for two hours before they are done.

If your apples are soggy, it is probably because they were cut too thick to start with. Make your slices as thin as you can possibly make them. I like to let the slicing attachment on my food processor do the job for me. That makes prep time mere minutes.

Preheat the oven to 200°F. Line 2 rimmed baking sheets with parchment paper to ensure the apples don't stick to the pan.

Core and thinly slice the apples about ⅛ inch thick with a mandoline, sharp knife, or the slicing attachment for your food processor. Arrange the slices in a single layer on the baking sheets. In a small bowl, combine the sugar and cinnamon. Sprinkle evenly over the apple slices.

Bake in the top and bottom third of the oven until the apples are dry and crisp, about 2 hours. Remove from the oven and let the apples cool completely before transferring to an airtight container for up to 3 days.

73 calories | 0.2 g fat | 0 g saturated fat | 19.5 g carbohydrates
14.8 g sugar | 0.3 g protein | 3.3 g fiber | 1 mg sodium

Refrigerator Pickled Carrots

1 pound carrots or baby carrots

½ cup rice vinegar (seasoned or unseasoned)

1 tablespoon sugar

1 tablespoon salt

¼ teaspoon caraway seed

½ teaspoon coarsely crushed black peppercorns (optional)

¼ cup finely chopped fresh flat-leaf parsley leaves (optional)

The title for the post in which this popular Snack Girl recipe appeared is "How to Use Up Old Carrots." You know those limp carrots that are hanging out in the bottom of your fridge? Take them out, peel and slice them, and do a refrigerator pickle.

I'm not suggesting you get out the canning jars. Add carrot sticks to some water, vinegar, and spices and leave in your fridge for twenty-four hours. This recipe is salty, sour, and sweet and will perk up those aging carrots.

Commercial cucumber pickles have on average 600 milligrams of sodium in one medium pickle. These carrots are also high in sodium because salt is a major component of the pickling process. You shouldn't munch on these all day like plain carrot sticks.

I use rice vinegar because it has a sweeter taste than regular vinegar. You can find it next to the Asian foods in your supermarket. If you don't have caraway seeds or black peppercorns, use another combination of dried spices that you like such as oregano, basil, or fennel seeds. You can also get a "pickling spice" mix in your supermarket's spice section.

These are great served sliced in a salad or next to a sandwich, just like a cucumber pickle.

Peel the carrots and cut into ¼-inch sticks about 4 inches long. If you are using baby carrots you can skip this step.

Pour 1½ cups water and the rice vinegar into a medium saucepan. Mix in the sugar, salt, caraway seed, and pepper, if using, and bring to a boil. Cook until the sugar and salt dissolve, about 1 minute.

Add the carrots and parsley (optional). Cool to room temperature and transfer to a storage container. These can be stored in the fridge for up to 1 month.

---

20 calories | 0.1 g fat | 0 g saturated fat | 3.5 g carbohydrates | 2.1 g sugar | 0.3 g protein
0.8 g fiber | 458 mg sodium

Greek Nachos

2 small whole-wheat pita rounds

½ tomato

½ cucumber

¼ cup crumbled feta cheese

**2 tablespoons prepared hummus,
or make your own (page 245)**

The whole concept of nachos is a wonderful one. You get a layer of crispy, a layer of melty, a layer of meaty and/or beany, and (if you are lucky) a layer of salad.

As a college student, I would buy a bag of chips, a packet of grated cheese, and a can of refried beans and call it dinner. This was a ridiculously easy meal but not the healthiest choice.

These nachos give you all the layers but emphasize the salad layer, which can be the best part if you give it a chance.

For the chips, buy the small rounds of 100 percent whole-wheat pita bread. Two rounds have 140 calories.

Preheat the oven to 375°F. Cut the pita rounds into quarters and pull apart the bread so that you have 8 triangles from each pita. Spread the bread on a baking sheet in one layer. Toast in the oven for 8 to 10 minutes.

While the bread is toasting, chop the tomato and cucumber and put them in a small bowl. Add the feta cheese and mix.

Put the toasted pita on a plate and drop some hummus in several spots on the chips. Spoon on the tomato mixture and serve.

---

157 calories | 6.2 g fat | 3.0 g saturated fat | 19.6 g carbohydrates | 3.4 g sugar | 7.4 g protein
3.9 g fiber | 420 mg sodium

Zucchini, Potato, and Egg Pie

Serves 4, ¼ pie per serving

---

1 teaspoon extra-virgin olive oil

1 small zucchini, grated (about 1¼ cups)

¼ cup chopped onion

1 cup frozen shredded potatoes, thawed

2 ounces water-packed roasted peppers, chopped

½ teaspoon smoked paprika

¼ teaspoon dried thyme

Salt and pepper to taste

4 large eggs

1 ounce grated Cheddar cheese (about ¼ cup)

Don't you love the word "pie"? It conjures an image of a grandmother with flour on her hands. This pie is more like a Spanish tortilla or baked omelet, and doesn't use flour at all.

This tastes good at room temperature and can be made ahead for a healthy lunch or snack.

You can find frozen raw shredded potatoes in your grocer's freezer section next to the hash browns. Sometimes called "country potatoes," they are simply potatoes that have been peeled and shredded for ease of use.

The jars of water-packed roasted red peppers are near the canned tomatoes or other canned vegetables. They are very low in calories and provide a lot of flavor. I like to use them in salads to add a burst of color when it isn't tomato season.

Heat a large nonstick ovenproof frying pan over medium heat. Heat the oil, then add the zucchini, onion, potatoes, and peppers. Cook for 5 minutes, turning the vegetables occasionally, until softened and starting to brown. Season with paprika, thyme, and salt and pepper. The vegetables should be well seasoned but not too salty.

While the vegetables are cooking, crack the eggs into a medium bowl and beat with a fork until combined—about 30 seconds. Add the cooked vegetables to the eggs and stir for 30 seconds to mix. Pour the egg mixture back into the pan. Use a spatula to make an even layer and top with grated cheese. Heat your broiler to high while the pie cooks. Cook the pie for 7 to 10 minutes, until the bottom of the pie has browned (lift the edge with a spatula to check).

To cook the top of the pie, place under the broiler for 2 minutes. Slide the pie onto a cutting board to cool.

This can be served hot, cold, or at room temperature.

---

140 calories | 8.1 g fat | 3.1 g saturated fat | 9.0 g carbohydrates | 2.3 g sugar | 8.6 g protein
1.6 g fiber | 145 mg sodium

Bake and Take Granola

Makes 2 cups,
¼ cup per serving

---

1 cup rolled oats (not instant)

**½ cup coconut flakes, sweetened
or unsweetened**

½ cup sliced almonds

¼ cup unsweetened applesauce

2 tablespoons dark brown sugar

2 teaspoons vanilla extract

1 teaspoon ground cinnamon

This granola is perfect for an on-the-go snack; it doesn't need milk or yogurt to enhance the flavor. A quarter cup is all you need to be satisfied, but you will want to eat more because it is so delicious.

You can omit the sugar, but be aware that the granola won't be as crunchy without it. Sweetened coconut flakes already have sugar. You can find unsweetened coconut in most health food stores and some supermarkets (like Whole Foods).

Add raisins or other dried fruit after you make the granola for added sweetness and flavor.

I use parchment paper for this recipe because I find that the granola will stick to aluminum foil or the baking sheet.

Preheat the oven to 375°F. Line a rimmed baking sheet with parchment paper. Mix the oats, coconut, almonds, applesauce, brown sugar, vanilla, and cinnamon in a large bowl. Spread onto the baking sheet. Bake for 10 minutes, remove from the oven, and stir. Bake for another 10 minutes or until lightly browned and crunchy.

Let cool for 10 minutes, then portion into small plastic bags or storage containers. As long as the container is sealed, the granola will last for 2 weeks at room temperature.

FOR GRANOLA USING SWEETENED COCONUT

108 calories | 4.9 g fat | 1.6 g saturated fat | 13.9 g carbohydrates | 5.3 g sugar

2.7 g protein | 2.4 g fiber | 14 mg sodium

Homemade Kettle Corn

Serves 3,
1 ½ cups per serving

¼ cup unpopped popcorn

1 tablespoon maple syrup

1 tablespoon chunky peanut butter (can substitute smooth)

Dash of salt

The cheapest and healthiest whole-grain snack you can make is popcorn. If you purchase a bag of popcorn kernels (usually found in the produce section of your supermarket), you will pay ten cents per serving. This is much less expensive than the bagged and flavored microwave variety.

My favorite way to make popcorn is to use the "el cheapo" microwave bag method. It turns out that you don't have to add anything (like oil) to popcorn to make it pop. Here is what you do:

1. Put ¼ cup popcorn in a brown paper bag. Fold the top over a few times and tape it.
2. Place in the microwave folded side up and cook on high for 2 to 3 minutes or until the pops are 5 seconds apart.

That's it! You can also just put the popcorn in a microwave-safe bowl tightly wrapped with plastic wrap and a few holes punched in it for ventilation. Who knew?

This is my favorite "watching the NFL when I should be cleaning" popcorn recipe. Be sure to bring some napkins with you because this gets messy. One of my friends eats this with a spoon.

Pop the popcorn in a microwave, an air popper, or on the stove. In a small bowl in the microwave, heat the maple syrup and peanut butter for 30 seconds. Mix with a spoon.

Put the popcorn in a large bowl and pour the warmed maple syrup and peanut butter over it. Add a dash of salt and mix with your hands until combined. Serve immediately.

102 calories | 3.4 g fat | 0.6 g saturated fat | 18.4 g carbohydrates | 4.5 g sugar
3.1 g protein | 3.0 g fiber | 25 mg sodium

Dips

Dips are essential to healthy eating because they make raw vegetables palatable. Of course, some of you eat raw veggies all day without dip, and I applaud you. However, I love to dip my carrots, celery, and bell pepper slices into something and so do my kids.

But do not think of the next three recipes exclusively as RVD (Raw Vegetable Delivery) devices. Think of them as sandwich spreads, whole-wheat pasta sauces, or roasted vegetable toppings. I don't know if I would mix these into any smoothies, but I would use them to flavor most of my savory food.

Homemade hummus and eggplant garlic dip are in line with the Mediterranean diet. Both recipes use natural peanut butter instead of tahini (sesame paste) because it is less expensive and easier to find. If you are allergic to peanut butter, you can use almond butter or tahini. Also, I used very little or no olive oil to flavor them, which is a big departure from the original recipes. Honestly, I don't think you'll notice.

Homemade Hummus

Makes 4 cups,
¼ cup per serving

Hummus is easy to make if you have a food processor or blender and you will save yourself some money by not buying it at the store.

1 or 2 garlic cloves

2 (15-ounce) cans chickpeas (garbanzo beans), drained (reserve ½ cup liquid from the cans) and rinsed

¼ cup extra-virgin olive oil

¼ cup creamy natural peanut butter (or almond butter)

½ lemon, or more to taste

Salt and pepper (optional)

Using a food processor, chop the garlic into small pieces. Add the beans, reserved bean liquid, olive oil, and peanut butter. Squeeze the lemon half into the rest of the ingredients. Blend until smooth and adjust the flavors with salt and pepper or more lemon juice.

115 calories | 5.8 g fat | 0.9 g saturated fat
13.0 g carbohydrates | 0 g sugar | 3.7 g protein
2.6 g fiber | 178 mg sodium

Eggplant Garlic Dip

Eggplant provides a ton of nutrients for very few calories. You cannot go wrong eating eggplant unless you soak it in olive oil. Eggplant acts like a sponge, so fried eggplant (while delicious) is a bit heavy on the calories.

This recipe is based on the classic eggplant dip baba ganoush.

Serves 3,
¼ cup per serving

1 small eggplant
(1 pound or less)

1 garlic clove

½ lemon, or more to taste

1 tablespoon creamy
natural peanut butter
(or almond butter)

Salt and pepper to taste

Preheat the oven to 450°F. Line a rimmed baking sheet with aluminum foil and slice the eggplant in half lengthwise. Place on the sheet cut side down and poke all over with a fork. Bake for 20 minutes or until the skin is blackened.

When the eggplant is cool, scoop the flesh from the skin and place in a food processor or blender. Add the garlic. Squeeze the lemon half into the food processor bowl and add the peanut butter, salt, and pepper. Blend until smooth. Taste and adjust the flavors with more lemon juice or salt and pepper.

69 calories | 3.0 g fat | 0 g saturated fat | 10.1 g carbohydrates
4.1 g sugar | 2.9 g protein | 5.5 g fiber | 100 mg sodium

Tuna Avocado Dip

Serves 4,
½ cup per serving

---

1 medium ripe avocado

1 (5-ounce) can chunk white albacore tuna packed in water, drained

1 small tomato, chopped

2 tablespoons fresh lemon juice

2 tablespoons prepared horseradish

Can you afford sushi for lunch every day? Neither can I. But you can make this dip and get some of the same flavors for less.

The tuna and avocado mixed together are heavenly. I add prepared horseradish, which you can usually find near the cottage cheese and sour cream in your local grocery store. It has almost zero calories and packs some heat, like wasabi.

Peel and pit the avocado and mash in a small bowl. Add the tuna, tomato, lemon juice, and horseradish and mix well.

---

120 calories | 7.7 g fat | 1.1 g saturated fat

6.7 g carbohydrates | 1.7 g sugar | 7.8 g protein

4.2 g fiber | 158 mg sodium

Desserts

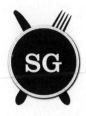

No-Bake Cookie Balls

Cookies done yet?

—Cookie Monster

You never have to sit and wait for your timer to go off if you make one of these four cookie recipes.

My kids love playing with Play-Doh, so these are a perfect afterschool snack for us to make together. Add them to your lunch box, have them with your coffee, or bring them to a potluck.

If you bring them to a party, it is fun to serve them in paper mini muffin cups to dress them up.

I store no-bake cookies in the refrigerator because they hold together better when they are cold. They will last about a week in a well-sealed container.

The first two recipes feature dates and almonds. Pitted dates are sweet and sticky; you can find them next to the raisins and prunes in your produce or baking section. Medjool dates are the perfect type, but if your store doesn't stock them, you can use whatever is available.

Almonds are a great alternative to butter in these recipes; they have much less of the saturated fat that most of us are trying to avoid. Most packaged almonds are dry roasted, which are perfect for these recipes. Do not buy salted or raw almonds, which are clearly labeled on the package.

The second two recipes feature quick oats as a replacement for wheat flour. Quick oats are simply more finely milled whole oats. If you have regular oatmeal in your pantry, just pulse it in a food processor a couple of times and you will produce quick oats.

Be sure to take out a plate for serving these before you start making them because your hands will be covered with cookie mixture, which you do not want to spread on your kitchen cabinets.

No-Bake Brownie Balls

Makes 20 balls,
1 (½-ounce) ball per serving

1 cup roasted almonds

15 pitted dates

²⁄₃ cup unsweetened cocoa
powder

1 tablespoon honey, maple syrup,
or agave syrup

Confectioner's sugar (optional)

Have a serving plate ready near your work area. Pulse the almonds in a food processor until ground. Add the dates, cocoa powder, honey, and 2 tablespoons water. Pulse until the mixture looks like bread crumbs. It will not clump into a single mass like other cookie doughs. Instead, it will be in soft pellets and will hold together when you press it.

Put a tablespoon of confectioner's sugar (if using) on a plate. With clean hands, scoop 2 teaspoons of dough into your palm and roll it into a ball (you may need a few drops more water to get the perfect consistency). Roll the ball in the sugar and set aside on your serving plate. Repeat until you have used all the dough.

Serve right away or refrigerate in a covered container for up to 1 week.

56 calories | 2.8 g fat | 0 g saturated fat | 8.5 g carbohydrates
5.4 g sugar | 1.7 g protein | 2.0 g fiber | 1 mg sodium

No-Bake Lemon Balls

**Makes 20 balls,
1 (½-ounce) ball per serving**

---

1 cup roasted almonds

2 lemons

1 cup pitted dates

**½ cup shredded coconut,
preferably unsweetened**

It is harder to find unsweetened shredded coconut than sweetened in the baking section of your store. However, I prefer to use it in this recipe; the lemon balls taste better with less sugar added because the dates are so sweet. You can find unsweetened coconut in health food stores, Whole Foods, and on the Internet.

Have a serving plate ready near your work area. Coarsely chop the almonds in a food processor. Roll the lemons against the counter to soften them, then juice with a hand juicer or citrus reamer into a small bowl. Remove the seeds from the juice and add the juice and dates to the food processor. Blend until a soft dough forms.

Put the coconut in a small bowl. With clean hands, scoop 2 teaspoons of dough into your palm and roll it into a ball (you may need to add a few drops of water to get the perfect consistency). Roll the ball in the coconut and set aside on the serving plate. Repeat until you have used all the dough.

Serve right away or refrigerate in a covered container for up to 1 week.

---

53 calories | 3.3 g fat | 0 g saturated fat | 4.9 g carbohydrates
3.4 g sugar | 1.1 g protein | 1.0 g fiber | 7 mg sodium

No-Bake Peanut Butter Balls

**Makes 15 balls,
1 (½-ounce) ball per serving**

---

1 cup quick oats

**½ cup smooth peanut butter (or
almond or cashew butter)**

2 tablespoons maple syrup

**Shredded coconut, sweetened or
unsweetened, or unsweetened
cocoa powder (optional)**

Have a serving plate ready near your work area. Put the quick oats in a medium bowl and mix in the peanut butter, maple syrup, and 2 tablespoons water. With clean hands, mix the dough until well blended. Scoop 2 teaspoons of dough into your palm and roll it into a ball (you may need a few drops more water to get the perfect consistency). Roll the ball in the coconut or cocoa powder (if using) and set aside on the plate. Repeat until you have used all the dough.

Serve right away or refrigerate in a covered container for up to 1 week.

WITHOUT COCONUT OR COCOA POWDER

78 calories | 4.7 g fat | 1.0 g saturated fat | 7.2 g carbohydrates
2.4 g sugar | 2.9 g protein | 1.1 g fiber | 40 mg sodium

No-Bake Pumpkin, Raisin, Oatmeal Balls

**Makes 12 balls,
1 (½-ounce) ball per serving**

1 cup quick oats

¼ cup raisins

1 teaspoon pumpkin pie spice

⅓ cup canned pumpkin puree

1 teaspoon vanilla extract

3 tablespoons honey

This recipe calls for ⅓ cup canned pumpkin. Use the rest of the pumpkin to make Pumpkin Overnight Pancakes (page 126).

Have a serving plate ready near your work area. In a medium bowl, combine the oats, raisins, and pumpkin pie spice. Add the pumpkin, vanilla, and honey. With clean hands, mix the ingredients until well blended. Scoop 2 teaspoons of dough into your palm and roll it into a ball (you may need to add a few drops of water to get the perfect consistency). Repeat until you have used all the dough.

Serve right away or refrigerate in a covered container for up to 1 week.

55 calories | 0.5 g fat | 0.1 g saturated fat | 12 g carbohydrates
6.4 g sugar | 1.1 g protein | 1.0 g fiber | 51 mg sodium

Almond Cookies

You can make these cookies in no time with a food processor. I love to serve them as a gluten-free Christmas cookie. They are a bit sticky to handle, but don't let that put you off.

Almonds are high in vitamin E, manganese, and magnesium, so you get a sweet dessert with some health benefits.

**Makes 16 cookies,
1 per serving**

1 cup blanched almonds,
whole or slivered,
plus 16 whole almonds

⅓ cup sugar

1 egg white

¼ teaspoon almond extract

Preheat the oven to 350°F. Line a cookie sheet with parchment paper.

In a food processor, process the cup of almonds and the sugar until very finely ground. Add the egg white and almond extract and pulse until the mixture forms a ball of dough.

Divide the dough into 4 sections. With clean hands, roll each section into 4 balls (making 16 cookies) and place on the parchment paper. Stick 1 almond into each cookie, pressing down so the almond stays put.

Bake for 15 minutes or until the cookies just start to turn golden.

60 calories | 3.7 g fat | 0 g saturated fat | 5.8 g carbohydrates
4.5 g sugar | 1.8 g protein | 0.9 g fiber | 4 mg sodium

Chocolate and Dried Cherry Bites

The results of this easy recipe look like you spent much more time in the kitchen than you did. I love the combination of cherries and chocolate.

**Makes 15 cookies,
1 per serving**

15 frozen mini fillo pastry shells

¼ cup bittersweet chocolate
chips

¼ cup dried cherries

Heat the oven to 350°F. Place the fillo shells on an ungreased baking sheet and fill each with 2 or 3 chocolate chips and 1 dried cherry. After the oven has come to temperature, turn it off and put in the baking sheet. After 5 minutes remove the bites from the oven. The chocolate will have melted a bit and the shells should be crisp. Cool and serve.

39 calories | 1.3 g fat | 0.6 g saturated fat | 6.2 g carbohydrates
3.0 g sugar | 0.6 g protein | 0 g fiber | 12 mg sodium

Mini Pecan Pies

**Makes 15 pies,
1 per serving**

15 frozen mini fillo pastry shells

1 large egg white

3 tablespoons brown sugar (not packed)

½ tablespoon butter, melted

¼ teaspoon vanilla extract

½ cup chopped pecans

A single slice of traditional pecan pie will cost you more than 500 calories, 37 grams of fat, and 26 grams of sugar. It makes the list of top ten holiday foods that you shouldn't eat, along with eggnog and creamed spinach. The thing is, pecan pie is delicious! Who doesn't love the combination of nuts, butter, sugar, and pastry? This miniature version hits all the right flavor notes without making your pants tighter. They're great for bake sales or holiday events. I love to have one with my afternoon coffee.

Preheat the oven to 375°F. Place the fillo shells on an ungreased baking sheet.

Mix the egg white, brown sugar, butter, vanilla, and pecans in a medium bowl until combined. Spoon into the fillo shells and bake for 10 to 15 minutes, until the shells are lightly browned.

Cool completely and serve, or store in a plastic container at room temperature for up to 1 week.

61 calories | 3.9 g fat | 0.5 g saturated fat | 6.2 g carbohydrates
1.9 g sugar | 1.5 g protein | 0.4 g fiber | 22 mg sodium

Revamped Chocolate Cake Mix Cupcakes

**Makes 18 cupcakes,
1 per serving**

**1 box chocolate cake mix such
as Betty Crocker Super Moist
Chocolate Fudge**

**8 ounces 2% or 0% fat
Greek yogurt**

1 large egg

Who doesn't love cupcakes? You don't have to share and they provide automatic portion control.

If you have ever been in a hurry to make a dessert for a potluck or bake sale, you have used a cake mix to make your cupcakes. I have a stash of cake mixes for emergencies and I will use them when necessary. No guilt here, especially since I figured out how to make them healthier.

Usually, you add water, vegetable oil, and eggs to the dry mix to make the batter. The half cup of vegetable oil adds 964 calories and not much flavor, but does make the cake moist. I looked for a lighter replacement and found Greek yogurt. With Greek yogurt, you get some protein with the fat, and a cup adds only 170 calories. You just saved almost 800 calories!

I use a Betty Crocker Super Moist Chocolate Fudge cake mix for these cupcakes. You can use any chocolate cake mix that you prefer. (I have not tried this upgrade for gluten-free mixes.)

I use foil wrappers because the cupcakes don't stick to them, unlike paper.

Preheat the oven to 325°F. Line a 12-cup and a 6-cup muffin tin with foil or paper liners. If you only have 12-cup tins, place 1 tablespoon water in the empty wells to keep the tin from burning or warping.

In a large bowl, beat the cake mix, yogurt, egg, and ½ cup water with a fork until well blended. There will still be lumps in the batter. Fill each muffin cup halfway with batter and bake for 18 to 23 minutes, until a toothpick inserted in the center of a cupcake comes out clean.

---

99 calories | 1.4 g fat | 0.6 g saturated fat | 21.5 g carbohydrates | 11.3 g sugar | 2.8 g protein
0.6 g fiber | 232 mg sodium

Birthday Carrot Cake

Serves 12

Nonstick spray

½ cup raisins

2 cups white whole-wheat flour

⅓ cup (packed) brown sugar

1 teaspoon baking powder

1 teaspoon baking soda

½ teaspoon ground cinnamon

½ teaspoon ground nutmeg

¼ teaspoon salt

1 ripe banana, mashed

¾ cup whole milk

1 large egg

1 teaspoon vanilla extract

2 large carrots, peeled and grated
(10 ounces, or about 2 cups)

½ cup chopped walnuts
(optional)

Coconut Frosting (page 264)
(optional)

Many readers have asked me for a healthier version of birthday cake. This moist and delicious carrot cake is made with raisins and mashed banana along with much less sugar than in a traditional cake. I swapped whole-wheat flour for the white flour, and I skipped the frosting. If you must have frosting (and who doesn't love frosting), check out my Coconut Frosting (page 264).

Walnuts are a tasty addition here and a nutritional powerhouse, but if you want to avoid the extra calories, omit them.

Position a rack in the center of the oven. Preheat the oven to 350°F. Spray a 9-inch round cake pan with nonstick spray. Soak the raisins in 1 cup warm water for about 5 minutes to soften them.

Mix the flour, sugar, baking powder, baking soda, cinnamon, nutmeg, and salt in a large bowl to combine. Add the banana, milk, egg, and vanilla, mixing until combined. Drain the raisins and stir into the batter along with the carrots and the walnuts, if using.

Pour the batter into the cake pan and spread it out to the edges. Bake until lightly browned and a toothpick inserted in the center comes out clean, about 35 minutes. Let the cake cool for a few minutes, then turn it out onto a wire rack to cool completely.

When fully cooled, top with frosting if desired.

WITHOUT FROSTING AND WALNUTS

131 calories | 1.4 g fat | 0 g saturated fat | 27.2 g carbohydrates | 10.8 g sugar
4.1 g protein | 2.9 g fiber | 73 mg sodium

WITH WALNUTS AND WITHOUT FROSTING

163 calories | 4.4 g fat | 0.6 g saturated fat | 27.7 g carbohydrates | 10.9 g sugar
5.3 g protein | 3.2 g fiber | 73 mg sodium

Coconut Frosting

Makes frosting for a 9-inch round cake or 8 cupcakes, 2 teaspoons per cupcake

---

¼ cup virgin coconut oil

¼ cup confectioner's sugar

¼ teaspoon vanilla extract

Can you have a cupcake without any frosting? Yes! You can always sprinkle some powdered sugar on the top to get a frosting-like effect.

Most people love cupcakes because of the frosting. I have tried a bunch of variations of this buttery concoction to try to get a lighter version that tastes yummy, is easy to make, and is stable at room temperature.

The problem is that the most beloved frosting is a buttercream: butter and confectioner's sugar beaten into a fluffy spread with a mixer. I have found it impossible to lighten this without dire consequences for the flavor, texture, or both.

I decided to toss out the butter and try virgin coconut oil, which you can find in the natural foods section of your store.

Virgin coconut oil is milder, sweeter, and richer tasting than butter and has a light texture. It is solid when cold, and liquefies at 76°F. Though it contains saturated fat, it is not the same type of saturated fat found in butter. Some research indicates that the saturated fat in virgin coconut oil is better for you than that found in animal products.

But coconut oil is still a fat, so you need to use it sparingly. What I love about coconut oil is that I don't have to get out my mixer to make frosting. I just blend it in a bowl and I get spreadable icing. Try using 2 teaspoons of icing per cupcake; I bet you will find that you don't need more.

If you hate the frosting, use the coconut oil on your skin (without the sugar). It is a great natural skin moisturizer.

Beat the coconut oil, confectioner's sugar, and vanilla in a small bowl with a fork or hand mixer until the consistency is smooth. This may take a few minutes of intense work.

Frost your favorite cake or cupcakes.

---

74 calories | 6.8 g fat | 5.9 g saturated fat | 3.8 g carbohydrates | 3.7 g sugar

0 g protein | 0 g fiber | 0 mg sodium

Apple Cake

Serves 16

Nonstick spray

1 box yellow cake mix, such as
Duncan Hines Yellow Cake Mix

1 cup unsweetened applesauce

2 tablespoons canola oil

2 teaspoons vanilla extract

1 teaspoon ground cinnamon

2 large eggs

2 large apples, peeled, cored,
and diced

There are those of us who love to bake and then there are people like me. I'm always in a hurry and I love the idea that I can make something for the latest bake sale from a box. In this recipe, I use unsweetened applesauce, which has only 50 calories per cup, to replace most of the oil. It totally works to keep the cake moist and adds a lovely apple flavor.

Preheat the oven to 350°F. Coat a 9 × 13 × 2-inch baking pan with nonstick spray.

In a large bowl, stir the cake mix, applesauce, canola oil, vanilla extract, cinnamon, and eggs until blended. Fold in the apples and pour into the prepared pan. Bake for 30 to 40 minutes, until a knife inserted into the center of the cake comes out clean.

189 calories | 6.2 g fat | 0.9 g saturated fat
31.4 g carbohydrates | 18.8 g sugar | 2.3 g protein
1.3 g fiber | 225 mg sodium

Healthier Apple Crisp

Serves 2,
½ cup per serving

---

1 medium apple, peeled, cored,
and chopped into ¼-inch pieces
(about 1 cup)

1 tablespoon brown sugar

1 tablespoon rolled or quick oats

½ teaspoon cinnamon

This recipe first appeared on my website, where it has been very popular. It's simple to make (the hardest part is peeling the apple), low in calories, and has all the flavors that make apple pie delicious. The apples cook down into a soft, creamy, pudding-like consistency so you might not notice the lack of butter in the recipe.

I will say that I did miss the butter when I first made these. If you miss it too, just add a little butter to each ramekin. You can make two small desserts in ceramic coffee mugs or ramekins, or just bake the apple mix in a small casserole dish. This recipe easily doubles for a family of four. I love using ramekins because they help me keep my portions the right size.

My daughter ate this dessert right up and my son hated it. Go figure.

Preheat the oven to 350°F. In a small bowl, mix the apples with the sugar, oats, cinnamon, and 1 tablespoon water and put in a small baking dish or 2 ramekins.

Bake for 15 minutes. Enjoy hot, cold, or at room temperature.

---

76 calories | 0.2 g fat | 0 g saturated fat | 19.2 g carbohydrates
13.9 g sugar | 0.4 g protein | 2.8 g fiber | 3 mg sodium

Instant Banana Pudding

Serves 1

1 ripe banana

10 raisins

¼ cup sweetened or unsweetened
shredded coconut

Dessert doesn't get much easier—or healthier—than this pudding, and it's a wonderful way to use up that overripe banana sitting on your counter. You don't need butter or cream, just a fork to mash a ripe banana into a sweet, sticky pudding.

Add raisins and coconut and you have a whole-food concoction that tastes like a decadent dessert. The difference is that the fat is from coconuts, not animals, and you get 7 percent of your daily value of iron from one serving.

This isn't particularly low in calories or sugar, but it is a great substitute for junk food.

In a small bowl, mash the banana with a fork or potato masher until it turns into a thick liquid. Spread the banana on a small plate and sprinkle with raisins and coconut.

218 calories | 7.2 g fat | 6.1 g saturated fat
41.2 g carbohydrates | 1.0 g sugar | 2.5 g protein
6.3 g fiber | 280 mg sodium

Upside-Down Sundae

Serves 1

1 cup sliced strawberries, fresh or frozen (thawed), or mango, blueberries, or raspberries

¼ cup slow-churned vanilla ice cream such as Edy's Slow Churned Vanilla Bean

1 teaspoon chocolate syrup

This sundae is upside down because, instead of ice cream with a few strawberry slices, you get strawberries with a little bit of ice cream.

When you measure out your ice cream and chocolate sauce, you will be surprised at how little you need to be satisfied. Even if you ate two of these sundaes (I dare you), you would still inhale only 226 calories. Compare that to the calorie bombs at your local restaurant or ice cream chain. For example, Chili's serves a Brownie Sundae that has 1,340 calories. When you start adding brownies to ice cream, things can get out of hand.

You can use either fresh or frozen fruit. If using frozen fruit, be sure to thaw it before you make your sundae. Isn't it nice to know that you ate a cup of antioxidant-filled strawberries (or another of your favorite fruits) as a dessert? Yay!

Put the strawberries, ice cream, and syrup in your favorite bowl and enjoy!

116 calories | 1.8 g fat | 1.1 g saturated fat
22.4 g carbohydrates | 16.4 g sugar | 2.6 g protein
2.1 g fiber | 27 mg sodium

Cinnamon, Vanilla, and Sugar Roasted Almonds

½ cup brown sugar

¼ teaspoon salt

1 teaspoon vanilla extract

1 tablespoon ground cinnamon

1 large egg white

2 cups almonds

These sweet and crunchy roasted almonds have good stuff like fiber and protein and taste like dessert. They are one of my favorite treats to have around the house because they have this lovely crunch and I feel less guilty when indulging in them. These are also great to give away as a holiday gift because they keep for a long time in an airtight container.

You can find unsalted roasted almonds in your produce section next to the walnuts and cashews. Be sure to use parchment paper (found next to the aluminum foil) on the baking sheet or you will need to use a power tool to get these almonds off the pan; they turn into a peanut brittle type of confection. Also, it takes a little work to break these apart after they're baked.

A serving here is 1 ounce, or about 23 almonds. Pack them in portion-controlled containers to take to work.

These are great for your afternoon coffee break.

Preheat the oven to 250°F. Line a rimmed baking sheet with parchment paper.

Mix together the brown sugar, salt, vanilla, and cinnamon in a medium bowl.

Beat the egg white and 1 tablespoon water in a small bowl until bubbles form and the egg white is broken up a bit. Pour in almonds and stir to coat them with the egg.

Add the almonds to the brown sugar mixture and mix well with your hands or a spoon. Spread the almonds on the baking sheet in a single layer.

Bake for 70 to 80 minutes, until the sugar has caramelized and the almonds are roasted. Cool completely, then transfer the almonds to an airtight container. Store at room temperature for up to 1 month.

---

183 calories | 14 g fat | 1.1 g saturated fat | 10.8 g carbohydrates | 5.6 g sugar | 6.2 g protein
3.5 g fiber | 40 mg sodium

Hot, Thick, and Dark Chocolate Drink

Serves 1

---

6 ounces (¾ cup) unsweetened almond milk

2 tablespoons unsweetened cocoa powder, such as Hershey's Special Dark

1 tablespoon sugar

½ teaspoon vanilla extract

You know when you crave chocolate and nothing else will satisfy you? This is your go-to treat to immerse yourself in the goodness that is chocolate.

This drink uses unsweetened dark cocoa powder, which you can find in the baking section next to the other cocoa powders. It is thick because of the fiber in the cocoa powder. I find the texture to be very comforting. You will have to whisk it quite vigorously to get the cocoa powder to dissolve. If you have one of those battery-powered milk frothers, it is perfect for this job.

I use unsweetened almond milk because it has a nice nutty flavor and only 40 calories per cup. You won't miss the cow's milk because this drink is all about the chocolate.

TO PREPARE IN ONE LARGE MUG
(ABOUT 14 OUNCES)

Mix 2 tablespoons of the almond milk with the cocoa powder, sugar, and vanilla in a large mug. Pour the rest of the almond milk into the mug and heat in the microwave until hot. Stir until all the chocolate is dissolved.

TO PREPARE IN TWO SMALL MUGS
(ABOUT 8 OUNCES EACH)

Mix 2 tablespoons of the almond milk with the cocoa powder, sugar, and vanilla in a small mug. In another mug, heat the remaining almond milk in the microwave. When hot, pour the almond milk into the first mug. Stir until all the chocolate is dissolved.

---

108 calories | 3.6 g fat | 0 g saturated fat | 20.1 g carbohydrates | 13.1 g sugar

2.8 g protein | 4.3 g fiber | 130 mg sodium

Acknowledgments

Snack-Girl.com has been a labor of love for me and my husband. Without our readers, their visits, comments, and support, we would not have been able to have a successful business or book. Thank you, dear readers, for all of your kindness and for coming back again and again.

I would like to thank my agent, Carole Bidnick, for finding me in the haystack of food blogs. She convinced me to write a book proposal when I thought that was a silly idea, and I have found that I actually loved writing a book. I am grateful for her guidance and warmth.

My editor, Sydny Miner, has been so involved with the conception and creation of this book that it seems ridiculous to thank her as a contributor. This book is as much hers as it is mine, and I was thrilled every time she answered the phone or responded to an e-mail (many, many times) because she was so helpful and engaged.

The recipe section of this book was influenced by a dedicated team of testers. My mother and a group of wonderful women from the Thursday Club of South Amherst gave me invaluable advice on flavor and technique. My husband, Matt, also contributed a few recipes and was the first taster on all of the dishes.

Finally, I want to thank my wonderful friends and family. My daughter, Ruby (with her seemingly unlimited confidence), inspires me every day to believe in myself. My son, Alex, gives me lots of kisses and hugs. My husband and business partner, Matt, has been amazing throughout this process. He inspired, supported, and encouraged me. Thank you, Matt, for this gift.

Scan this QR code or visit www.snack-girl.com/rescuebonus to receive
additional recipes and helpful tips for your healthy journey.

Index